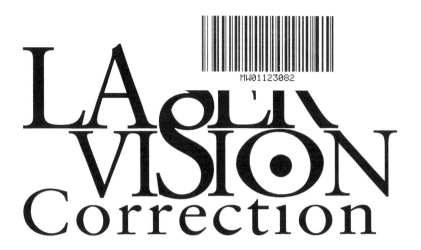

LASER VISION Correction

A New Age in Vision

LASER VISION
Correction

A New Age in Vision

HAROLD STEIN
M.D., FRCS (C)

RAYMOND STEIN
M.D., FRCS (C)

ALBERT CHESKES
M.D., FRCS (C)

Ethis Communications, Inc., New York, NY

Laser Vision Correction
A New Age in Vision

by
Harold A. Stein, MD, FRCS(C)
Raymond M. Stein, MD, FRCS(C)
Albert T. Cheskes, MD, FRCS(C)

Bochner Eye Institute
40 Prince Arthur Avenue
Toronto, Ontario M5R 1A9
Canada

For information concerning this title contact:
Bochner Eye Institute
40 Prince Arthur Avenue
Toronto, Ontario M5R 1A9
Canada
416-960-2020

Published by Ethis Communications, Inc.
258 West 99th Street, #2
New York, NY, 10025
USA

ISBN: 0-9666621-0-5

Library of Congress Catalog Card Number: 98-87243

Contents

Foreword vii

Acknowledgments viii

Preface ix

Chapter 1: A New Age in Vision 1

Chapter 2: Is Laser Vision Correction Right for You? 9

Chapter 3: The Eye and Vision 17

Chapter 4: Errors of Refraction 27

Chapter 5: Creating New Eyes:
            How Laser Vision Correction Works 37

Chapter 6: The Experience of PRK 45

Chapter 7: If You Have LASIK 55

Chapter 8: Alternatives to Laser Vision Correction 63

Chapter 9: The Decision Process 71

Chapter 10: Choosing a Refractive Surgeon 77

Chapter 11: Questions and Answers 85

Glossary 95

Index 98

Foreword

It is no coincidence that the first clinical text on the excimer laser*
was prepared by three Canadian authors, who were early users of an
American manufactured excimer system. While the U.S. Food and
Drug Administration (FDA) regulations in the United States restricted
the use of the excimer in the country of its invention to a limited
number of patients, the less rigid Canadian regulatory environment
allowed a more rapid appreciation and development of the clinical
value of the technology.

Canadian surgeons adopted excimer lasers to treat refractive errors with enthusiasm, none more so than those at the Bochner Eye
Institute in Toronto. Harold A. Stein, Albert T. Cheskes, and Raymond
M. Stein received their first laser system in September 1991. They
now have over 7 years of clinical experience with it, treating myopia,
astigmatism and hyperopia. The three authors of this book have worked
long and hard to meet the expectations of their patients.

This group has had substantial previous experience with refractive
surgery and is able to make a fair comparison between the results
that are obtained with the excimer laser and results using other refractive technologies. Much remains to be learned. The clinical work
of these Canadian surgeons has made the path to be followed less
difficult for all of us.

Stephen L. Trokel, MD
New York, NY
September 1998

Editor's Note: Dr. Stephen Trokel played a leading role in the invention of laser
vision correction techniques. He is currently professor of clinical ophthalmology at
Columbia University College of Physicians and Surgeons.

* Harold A. Stein, Albert T. Cheskes, and Raymond M. Stein: *The Excimer: Fundamentals and Clinical Use.* Thorofare, NJ, SLACK Incorporated, 1994. Second
edition, 1997.

Acknowledgments

We could not have produced this book without the help of many people. First and foremost we owe an enormous debt of gratitude to our patients. Their faith—especially in the early days—in our skills and our instruments has made our work possible. It is a source of pride and pleasure that we were able to reward that faith with good vision.

Similarly, we are indebted to the literally hundreds of surgeons, scientists, and engineers from around the world whose work has made laser vision correction a reality. Our early results were good; and our current results are even better. We owe this improvement to the ever-better instruments and techniques that these hard-working investigators have given us.

The staff of the Bochner Eye Institute makes our work possible. Without their skill, care, and dedication, none of our work would be possible. In particular, we want to thank Jill Klintworth, Robin Inrig, Lynn Maund, Linda Hargreaves, Peter Schilling, Ghani Salim, Sheffield Wong, and Margarida Morais for their loyalty and dedication to patient care.

David Kellner, David Rossman, and Farzad Sarmast helped in the preparation of the text. DeborahAnne Chingas Sandke of :DACS Design in New York, provided most of the drawings, as well as the overall design of the text. The cover design reflects the creative talents of Mr. Robert Shropshire of Mad Dog Communications.

Finally, we are grateful to our families for their patience, support and assistance, which allowed the writing of this book to go forward.

Harold Stein, MD, FRCS(C)
Raymond Stein, MD, FRCS(C)
Albert Cheskes, MD, FRCS(C)

Preface

After almost two decades of research and hundreds of millions of dollars in investment, laser vision correction has come of age. Once a revolutionary procedure, years of scientific study and the experience drawn from millions of successful procedures have brought laser vision correction into the mainstream of vision care. It is at last ready for "prime time."

This is truly a happy moment in vision care. For the first time ever, near- and farsighted people, and people with astigmatism, can get good functional vision without dependence on appliances like glasses or contact lenses.

What do we mean by "good functional vision"? Here's a fact: the ophthalmologists at the Bochner Eye Institute have done many thousands of cases; and, after their procedure, more than 98% of our laser vision correction patients can qualify for a driver's license without glasses or contact lenses. Before laser vision correction, almost none could have qualified. Many couldn't even see the eye chart!

For the first time, exciting new vistas are opening up to people who were previously hampered by the need to wear glasses or contact lenses. People who hate the way they look in glasses or are tired of the hassle of contact lenses now don't need them for the tasks of daily life. People who want to dive or water ski, or join in other active sports, can now do so without worry. All of a sudden, careers in aviation, the fire department, the police, or the military are open to people who could never before qualify! It's a new age.

We are proud to be a part of it. Our faith in the procedure led us to invest almost a million dollars in a vision correction laser in 1991, one of the first in Canada. We have been involved with the evolution of laser vision correction ever since. In fact, we were doing laser vision correction for years before the U.S. Food and Drug Administration (FDA) finally approved a laser for use in the U.S. It wasn't until 1996 that the FDA approved the laser that we had been using with excellent results since 1991!

We believe in the value of laser vision correction. That is why we do it every day. And that is why we wrote this book. We want people to know about this extraordinary procedure. But as good as laser vision correction is, it is not for everybody. The more you know about it, the better equipped you will be to decide whether it makes sense for you or someone you care about.

Harold A. Stein, MD, FRCS(C)
Raymond M. Stein, MD, FRCS(C)
Albert T. Cheskes, MD, FRCS(C)
Bochner Eye Institute
Toronto, Ontario

To our patients.

Your faith in us is a source of pride and an inspiration to us.

CHAPTER 1

A New Age in Vision

Eye doctors are lucky people. We spend our days restoring people's sight, and few activities are more satisfying than helping people see.

Today's ophthalmologists and optometrists are lucky for another reason: This is, we believe, the most exciting time ever in the history of vision care. Indeed, eye care professionals working today have witnessed not one but two revolutions. The first of these involved cataract surgery. Cataract removal, the most common form of eye surgery, used to be a major operation that left patients with thick glasses and poor vision. Thirty years ago, the only good thing you could say about cataract surgery was that it was better than the alternative, which was to go blind from cataracts.

In just one generation, cataract surgery has changed completely. Today, cataract removal is considered "minor" surgery. The actual operation can take less than 15 minutes. Patients walk in, have their operation, and go home a few hours later. Instead of having to wear thick, heavy "cataract glasses," a tiny lens is implanted in the patients' eyes, restoring them to excellent vision. For those of us who remember the "old" days, contemporary cataract surgery seems like a miracle.

A Second Revolution

The second revolution is laser vision correction. For the first time in history, we have a sophisticated yet straightforward and non-traumatic procedure that allows nearsighted and farsighted people, and people with astigmatism, to have good natural vision with little or no dependence on corrective lenses.

For many of us, laser vision correction is the most important and most exciting medical development of our lifetimes. Patients who, after almost a lifetime of dependence on glasses, finally experience good natural vision, often call laser vision correction a "miracle." We find it extremely satisfying to be involved with a procedure that is bringing dramatic and happy changes to our patients' lives.

Laser vision correction is the product of careful, exacting science. It is the fruit of years of hard work and hundreds of millions of dollars of research funding. Developed by eye surgeons, physicists, and engineers working together, laser vision correction is an example of medical science at its best.

Today's laser vision correction technologies have been proven in dozens of scientific research studies involving tens of thousands of patients. (These have been done at centers around the world.) Like all good research, the results of these studies have been published in the peer-reviewed scientific literature and are available for all to read.

Today, laser vision correction is an established technology that is in widespread use on every continent. More than 2 million successful procedures have already been done, and thousands more are being added to the total each day.

The Driving Force

What's fueling the rapid expansion of laser vision correction? Just one thing: word of mouth. People who have laser vision correction love it, and they tell their friends. Their friends then have laser vision correction and go on to tell *their* friends.

An ophthalmologist from the U.S., Kurt Buzard, MD, has talked about what he calls the "miracle factor" associated with laser vision correction. By that he means the sudden excitement at discovering what it is like to have good natural vision after years of wearing glasses or contact lenses. To patients, it is a miracle; and that inspires them to tell their friends, family, and coworkers about it.

Another U.S. ophthalmologist estimates that every person on whom he performs laser vision correction refers, on average, nine other people for examination and possible laser vision correction! Laser vision correction has a powerful and positive effect on people's lives. The excitement that laser vision correction generates in people who have had it is contagious.

A New Technology Solves Ancient Problems

Nearsightedness, farsightedness, and astigmatism are common problems that have plagued humankind from the dawn of time. Twenty years ago, there were two choices for dealing with those problems: glasses or contact lenses. Today's eye doctors have a third option: laser vision correction.

Compared to laser vision correction, glasses and contact lenses are "old technology." In addition, glasses and contact lenses are temporary "patches." While glasses and contact lenses help you see, they don't alter the underlying problem—the instant you take off your glasses or contact lenses, your vision problems return. Laser vision correction is fundamentally different: it literally gives you new eyes with which to see.

When we talk about glasses being "old technology," we mean really old. Eyeglasses date from the middle ages when monks first used clear crystals to help them read. Glasses have improved slowly since then; but the last fundamental advance in glasses technology was probably Benjamin Franklin's invention of the bifocal lens in the late 18th century.

Contact lenses are a more modern technology. Glass contact lenses were invented in the late 19th century, but only a few of them were made and used. Contact lenses didn't become practical until after World War II, when plastic contact lenses were developed. The real boom in contact lenses began in the 1970s, with the advent of soft lenses.

As its name implies, laser vision correction is dramatically different from glasses or contact lenses. Laser vision correction is a true 21st century technology, and it is quickly becoming obvious that laser vision correction will have more far-reaching effects than any other eyecare procedure developed in this century.

How Does It Work?

As we all know, the eye is an optical system that focuses light and allows us to see. Nearsightedness, farsightedness, and astigmatism are all the result of the eye's inability to focus light correctly. Both of the old technologies—glasses and contact lenses—correct the focussing problem by putting an additional lens in front of the eye. This added lens, whether a contact lens or a lens in a pair of glasses, helps the eye bring light to a focus.

Laser vision correction works on an entirely different principle. It changes the shape of the cornea, the clear dome through which light enters the eye. The cornea is not merely a transparent window, it also acts as a lens to focus light for the eye. Laser vision correction changes the shape of the cornea in very slight, very precise ways. By changing its shape, we alter the focussing power of the cornea. For example, in nearsighted people, the eye's optical system is too strong. A small change in the shape of the cornea can turn it into a slightly less powerful lens, correcting the eye's nearsightedness.

Just as each pair of glasses is custom-designed for a particular patient, with laser vision correction, each person's correction is custom-designed for that particular eye. The result is that people who are nearsighted, farsighted, or have astigmatism can see clearly without corrective lenses. Their vision is just like the vision of people who were born with good natural vision.

Russian Roots

It has been known for more than 100 years that changing the shape of the eye could enhance its ability to focus. What was missing was a technology that could quickly, accurately, and painlessly transform the shape of the eye. With the advent of the computer-controlled excimer laser, we have a tool that will do just that.

The first glimmerings that a practical procedure for changing the shape of the eye might be found came in 1978, when Russian ophthalmologist Svyatoslav Fyodorov reported the technique now called radial keratotomy—"RK" for short. RK was a simple surgical technique that helped nearsighted people see clearly.

RK involves making four or more tiny incisions in the cornea. These tiny incisions cause the cornea to flatten very slightly, changing its optical properties. This change in shape was just what nearsighted people needed in order to be able to see more clearly. RK works, but RK is only helpful in low-to-moderate nearsightedness, and there is nothing that RK can do that laser procedures can't also do. While some RK is still performed, it has largely been supplanted by laser vision correction.

Enter the Laser

Dr. Fyodorov's demonstration that a simple surgery could correct nearsightedness sparked an outpouring of research activity that continues to this day. (This use of surgery to correct vision problems is called *refractive surgery.*) Although RK worked, efforts began almost immediately to improve on it. In a burst of creativity, physicists and engineers worked with ophthalmic surgeons to develop lasers that could produce precise changes in the shape of the cornea. These efforts gave us laser vision correction. Today, laser vision correction is the most important branch of refractive surgery.

But laser vision correction isn't the only branch of refractive surgery. Another group of surgeons and scientists developed tiny plastic implants (called KeraVision Rings) that can be implanted within the cornea. These researchers are said to be working on "intracorneal"

"I'm delighted I did it."

NAME: Don Matthews
AGE: 59
OCCUPATION: Head Coach, Toronto Argonauts
PROCEDURE: PRK for myopia
OPHTHALMOLOGIST: Dr. Raymond Stein
BEFORE LASER VISION CORRECTION: 20/200
AFTER LASER VISION CORRECTION: 20/25

Don wore glasses and contact lenses all his adult life until undergoing PRK with Dr. Raymond Stein 2 years ago.

I heard about laser vision correction from my optometrist, and I had grown tired of the hassle of glasses and contact lenses. I figured that this advancement is safe and predictable, and I can take advantage of this incredible technology. So I decided to have it done and I'm delighted I did.

Don says he went into the procedure with "no nervousness," and that the discomfort he experienced afterwards was "minimal."

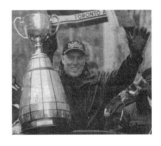

The procedure was explained to me very thoroughly, and I had no apprehension. It was very easy. I had it done 8 or 10 days before I went to training camp. That year, as head coach of the Toronto Argonauts football team, we captured the Grey Cup. It was great to be able to see the field without wearing glasses or contact lenses.

Don heartily recommends PRK to "anyone who qualifies."

My youngest son had it done because of the success I had. His vision was certainly as bad as mine was, if not worse, and he's now better than 20/20.

solutions, since their devices are implanted within the cornea.

A third group has pursued a technology derived from cataract surgery. These surgeons implant lenses within the eye to correct vision. We refer to these as *intraocular lenses.*

Like laser techniques, intraocular and intracorneal techniques have been shown to work. All three technologies are able to produce stable, predictable changes in the way the eye focuses. All of them can help people with vision problems see clearly.

The most successful (by far) of the new technologies has been laser vision correction. The laser's success results from its extraordinary precision and its versatility, as well as from the simplicity of the procedure. Intraocular and intracorneal solutions, while effective, are useful to correct a limited range of problems. The laser's range is much greater. For example, intraocular solutions are useful only for extreme nearsightedness or extreme farsightedness. These are very rare conditions. The laser corrects all of the "garden variety" eye conditions that one sees everyday, as well as many uncommon conditions.

Using excimer lasers, ophthalmologists are able to correct the cornea's shape with an accuracy undreamed of just a few years ago. These lasers use a cool beam of ultraviolet light to "ablate" (vaporize) tiny amounts of tissue from the surface of the eye. (We will discuss this in greater detail in subsequent chapters.) Controlled by computers, the new lasers leave behind an incredibly smooth surface that heals quickly and provides what the eye needs: a clear, smooth, properly-shaped optical surface.

The Future is Now

Today's laser vision correction procedure is amazingly brief. It takes no more than 20–30 minutes to treat *both* eyes; and most of that time is spent preparing for the laser treatment. The actual time in which the laser is working is likely to be 2 minutes or less (that's the total for both eyes).

Laser vision correction technology has come of age and is clearly ready for widespread application. There are laser vision centers staffed by well-trained ophthalmologists located around the world. But there is more capacity for laser vision correction than is currently being used. What's holding people back? In most cases it is simply lack of knowledge. Many people don't yet know about laser vision correction. Others know it exists but don't know that it can benefit them. Still others are worried about having a procedure—*any* procedure—

done to their eyes. Knowledge will help all of these people. Laser vision correction has proven safe and effective. We wrote this book to help readers understand precisely how laser vision correction works and why medical authorities have declared it both safe and effective.

Laser vision correction is a superb technology that is rapidly gaining wider acceptance. Every day, patients who have had laser vision correction tell us how much they enjoy their new natural vision. Still, there is no one technology that is right for everybody. Glasses work for some people. Contact lenses work for others. For others, the answer is laser vision correction. If you need vision correction, the choice is yours. The more you know about laser vision correction, the better equipped you will be to decide whether it's right for you.

CHAPTER 2

Is Laser Vision Correction Right for You?

Introduction

Laser vision correction has already helped more than two million people achieve good natural vision. These people have told their friends; and, as the word spreads, thousands of people are asking, "Is laser vision correction right for me?"

Although new, laser vision correction is rapidly becoming an accepted way of dealing with common vision problems. If you are nearsighted, farsighted, or have astigmatism, you may already be considering laser vision correction.

As physicians who were involved in the pioneering early efforts to find a better way than glasses to correct vision, we are happy to see that laser vision correction has come of age. Laser vision correction has joined glasses and contact lenses as a "mainstream" way of helping people see more clearly.

Now that the safety and effectiveness of laser vision correction have been demonstrated, nearsighted people, farsighted people, and those with astigmatism have a choice. Do they want glasses, contact lenses, or the potential of natural vision available through laser vision correction?

We think that is an important question, and it's worthwhile taking a little time to answer it carefully. Laser vision correction is a great opportunity; but like all opportunities, it is not right for everybody. There are three important factors that must be taken into account in deciding whether laser vision correction is right for you:

- Can laser vision correction help your particular vision problem?
- Do you have any other eye condition or general health problem that might interfere with laser vision correction?
- Will laser vision correction meet your personal needs?

Thinking Like a Doctor

If you were to come to one of us and ask, "Is laser vision correction right for me?" the first thing we would do is test your vision. Most people who wear glasses or contact lenses do so to correct nearsightedness, farsightedness, or astigmatism. The good news is that, except in extreme cases, nearsightedness, farsightedness, and astigmatism are treatable with laser vision correction. Your eye doctor will tell you whether your vision can be corrected by the new excimer laser technique.

Even if you are too near- or farsighted for laser vision correction, there is still good news. Other procedures are on the horizon that promise good natural vision for people who are poor candidates for laser vision correction. (See Table 1 for vision problems that can and can't be treated by laser vision correction.)

Health Issues

Once we know that your vision problem can be corrected by a laser procedure, we would want to ask some questions about your general health and examine your eyes. The purpose of this "history" and eye examination is to be sure that there is no condition that could interfere with getting a good result from laser treatment. For example, some autoimmune diseases—like rheumatoid arthritis and lupus—can disrupt the healing response and lead to an imperfect laser vision correction result. People with these conditions are often wisest to stay with their current mode of vision correction.

Other conditions, like very dry eyes, should be cleared up prior to surgery. (See Table 2 for conditions that may make it wise to postpone or cancel plans for laser vision correction.)

TABLE 1   What vision problems can laser vision correction treat?

Laser vision correction can treat:
>   Most nearsightedness (myopia)
>   Most farsightedness (hyperopia)
>   Most astigmatism

Laser vision correction isn't used to treat:
>   Extreme near- or farsightedness
>   Extreme degrees of astigmatism
>   Irregular astigmatism
>   Presbyopia

TABLE 2   Conditions that usually prevent or delay laser vision correction

Laser vision correction is usually not done if one of the following conditions exits:
> Autoimmune diseases, such as:
>> Lupus
>> Rheumatoid arthritis
> Cataracts (with loss of vision)
> Diabetic retinopathy
> Uncontrolled glaucoma
> Severe dry eye
> Large pupil size
> Under 18 years old

Conditions that may cause postponement of laser vision correction:
> Herpes infection of the eye
> Pregnancy
> Chronic eye infections
> Use of certain medications

Is It Right for You?

Let's assume that your eye doctor has determined that laser correction can help your vision and that your general and ocular health are fine. Now the ball is back in your court. It is time to consider your personal vision needs.

Because anything that affects your eyes is important, people considering laser surgery want to get all the facts. We urge all potential laser vision correction patients to gather facts, consider them carefully, and discuss the matter with friends and family. After all, your sight is a very precious gift. For many people, the decision to have laser vision correction is one of the most important decisions of their lives. We wrote this book to help patients make thoughtful, intelligent, well-informed decisions.

An Important Decision

We believe in laser vision correction. We believe that it is a wonderful procedure, a procedure that has given the gift of good vision to millions of people. As the years roll on, hundreds of millions of people will benefit from laser vision correction. If we didn't believe in it wholeheartedly, we wouldn't offer it to our patients, and we wouldn't have written this book! But apprehension about doing something to your eyes is completely natural. Becoming comfortable with laser vision correction means learning as much as you can about it. Our goal is to help you make a decision based on facts rather than fear.

Making the decision to have laser vision correction means becoming comfortable with an innovative idea: that a laser can gently reshape the surface of your eye to give you better vision. Most people want to share the task of learning with a family member or trusted friend. That's why, if you were a patient at the Bochner Eye Institute, we would invite you to have the friend or family member accompany you whenever you came to the center. After all, if someone is going to help you make a decision, that person should be as informed as you! If possible, your support person should be with you every step of the way.

For some people the decision process is swift. Others need time to get used to the idea. Knowledge will make the decision-making process easier. And if you decide to have laser vision correction, knowledge of what to expect will also make you more comfortable on the day of the procedure. We therefore urge you to learn all you can about laser vision correction.

What Can You Expect from Laser Vision Correction?

The key to satisfaction with laser vision correction is realistic expectations. The overwhelming majority of our patients achieve good, functional *uncorrected* distance vision. In technical terms (which we will explain in the next two chapters), this means 20/40 or better distance vision without glasses. How good is 20/40 vision? With 20/40 vision, it is safe and legal to drive—and to do all the other tasks of daily life—without glasses for distance vision.

After surgery a few patients use glasses for very demanding tasks—like long stretches of night driving—or to get the sharpest vision possible. But most don't need contact lenses or glasses for their normal routines. And they don't ever have to depend on finding their glasses in an emergency.

We talk in terms of distance vision because, unless you choose monovision (see Chapter 4), laser vision correction works primarily on correcting distance vision. Everybody experiences a loss of near vision as they approach and enter their 40s. This is a condition called *presbyopia*, and laser vision correction does not yet offer help for it. If your distance vision is fine, and you just need glasses for reading, laser vision correction is not likely to be your best option.

What laser vision correction potentially means is good natural dis-

"I don't need glasses or contact lenses anymore."

NAME:	Mark Hotz
AGE:	41
PROCEDURE:	PRK for myopia and astigmatism
OPHTHALMOLOGIST:	Dr. Albert Cheskes
BEFORE LASER VISION CORRECTION:	20/400
AFTER LASER VISION CORRECTION:	20/20

Mark cites "vanity" as the primary reason for choosing laser vision correction.

The outcome was quite successful. I don't need glasses or contact lenses anymore. As far as I'm concerned, if you have the money, you should do it. I would have spent two or three times the money. I'm that happy with it.

Mark considered laser vision correction for about a year before deciding to go to the Bochner Eye Institute for a consultation.

I was waiting for it to be on the market a bit longer to see if there were any long-term adverse effects, or medium-term effects, but I didn't hear of any. A friend of mine had it done by Dr. Cheskes. My friend is a very conservative type of person. I figured if he could do it then I could do it. Once I decided to do it, I was down there the next day.

Two years later, Mark is still happy with the results of the procedure.

My vision has been pretty stable, and I don't have to wear contacts or glasses. The only thing is that at dusk, it is a little more difficult to see than during the daytime. Except for that, I can see very clearly. I can see better than most people.

tance vision with little or no dependence on glasses or contact lenses.

Who Wants Laser Vision Correction?

Today, most of the people who have laser vision correction do so because they are dissatisfied with glasses and contact lenses. As time goes on and laser vision correction becomes "ordinary," we think this will change—people will choose laser vision correction because it makes their life so much simpler and better.

However, there are millions of people who are unhappy with glasses and contact lenses! Many spectacles wearers remember being teased about them as children or feel that wearing glasses gets in the way of an active lifestyle. For others, having to depend on glasses doesn't fit their image of themselves as self-reliant individuals, who don't need help with the basic routines of life.

Most laser vision correction patients have tried contact lenses. In many cases, they started out happy with contact lenses but ran into trouble with them. It is normal for eyes to get drier with age, and in many people this makes their contact lens wear less comfortable. In other cases, patients developed an allergic reaction to contact lens deposits or lens care solutions. Some develop blood vessels growing into the cornea. Whatever the reason, for some people contact lens wear becomes difficult or impossible—even after years of success.

Still others simply can't stand the hassle of contact lens care. Daily cleaning and disinfection take too much time from their busy lives. And contact lenses are an added burden when traveling or camping out.

The typical laser vision correction candidate, then, is someone who dislikes glasses and can't, or would prefer not to, wear contact lenses. Most often these are people with active lifestyles who find that glasses or contacts get in the way. Laser vision correction is particularly attractive to patients who enjoy swimming and other water sports.

Is Laser Vision for You?

The best candidates for laser vision correction are people with realistic expectations and a strong desire to lessen their dependence on glasses or contact lenses. Here are some questions that will help you determine whether you are good candidate for laser vision correction:

- Would you choose good vision that lets you drive and play sports without glasses over "perfect" vision with glasses?
- Do you think that you look better without glasses?

- Do allergies or dry eye affect your ability to wear contact lenses?
- Does discomfort limit the number of hours each day that you can wear contact lenses?
- Do you feel that glasses or contact lenses restrict your activities?
- Does having to wear glasses or contact lenses feel like a "handicap" to you?
- Is irritation from contact lenses, especially at the end of the day, a bother to you?
- Can you accept the possibility that you might need a second laser procedure to fine tune your vision?
- Would good vision without glasses be a satisfactory result for you even if that vision wasn't quite as good as your vision now with glasses?
- Is having good natural vision important enough to postpone other purchases?
- Is having to take care of contact lenses a hassle? Do you cut corners on contact lens care, even though you know it is safer not to?

People who answer "Yes" to questions like these are likely to get the maximum value from laser vision correction and be happiest with the results.

Having Realistic Expectations

It's important to have realistic expectations about laser vision correction. Laser vision correction can give good functional vision, either without glasses or with greatly reduced dependence on glasses. When glasses (or contacts) are needed after laser vision correction, it's often just for specific tasks like driving at night. Laser vision correction can end your dependence on glasses for the necessities of life, but there is no guarantee that after laser vision correction you will see as well without glasses as you now see with glasses.

Is this a concern for you? Here is a litmus test that can help you determine how you feel about this matter. See whether you agree with Jane, the subject of this brief story. Jane is 27 years old. Before laser vision correction she was nearsighted and, without glasses, had 20/600 vision (her prescription was –6.00). Without her glasses Jane couldn't read the clock, catch a ball, cook dinner, or even think about driving. But with glasses Jane could see 20/15. Then Jane had laser vision correction. Now Jane can see 20/25 without glasses; but wearing glasses doesn't help her see any better than that. She can swim, play tennis and volleyball, see the clock easily, drive, and lead a fully normal life—without ever wearing glasses. The only glasses Jane wears now are fashion sunglasses—with no prescription. She is thrilled. She thinks laser vision correction was one of the smartest things she ever did.

Most people are like Jane: they would much rather have good, functional vision without glasses than wear "Coke bottle" glasses to get 20/15 vision. But would you? Do you think that Jane was better off with thick glasses and excellent vision than she is with no glasses and good vision? If you are an absolute perfectionist about your vision and don't mind the discomfort of glasses or the inconvenience of contact lenses, talk to your vision professional about what is reasonable to expect from laser vision correction.

Doing What's Right for You

Does Jane's story appeal to you? Is it important to you to lessen your dependence on glasses or contact lenses? If so, laser vision correction may be just the right thing for you.

CHAPTER 3

The Eye and Vision

Introduction

Sight is our primary connection to the world. Naturally, our eyes, the organs that make sight possible, are very important to us. As scientists, the more we study the eye, the more impressed we are with its functionality, its resilience, and even its beauty.

In laser vision correction, we change the shape of the eye very

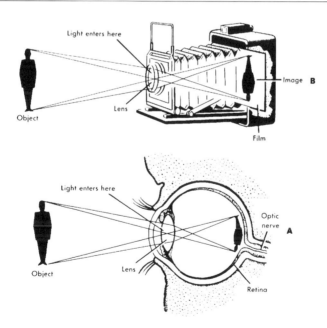

Figure 1 *The eye is like a camera. In both cases, light enters through a lens that focuses the light on a detection device. In the camera, a glass lens focuses the light on a piece of film or an electronic sensor (the detection device). In the eye, the cornea and crystalline lens act as the focusing system, and the retina is the device that picks up the focused image. (From Stein HA, Slatt BJ, Stein RM:* The Ophthalmic Assistant *ed 6. St. Louis, Mosby-Yearbook, 1994. Reprinted with permission.)*

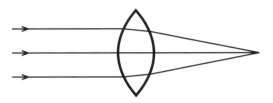

Figure 2 *A lens bends light rays to focus them at a point.*

slightly in order to enhance the way it focuses light. To understand how laser vision correction works, then, one must first understand how the eye works to focus light.

The Eye is Like a Camera

The eye can be likened to a modern digital camera, which has a lens in front to focus the light and a light sensor at the back that registers the focused image (Figure 1).

In the case of the eye, two structures, the *cornea* and the *crystalline lens*, correspond to the camera's lens. The *retina*, at the back of the eye, corresponds to the light sensor in a digital camera (or to the film in a traditional camera). After the eye's optical system has focused light on the retina, the retina registers the image and sends it via the optic nerve to the brain. The brain interprets the signals from the retina, giving us the perception that we know as sight.

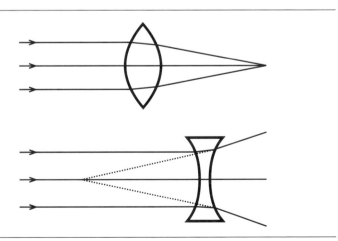

Figure 3 *A converging lens is convex in shape and brings light rays to a focus. A diverging lens is concave and causes light rays to spread apart.*

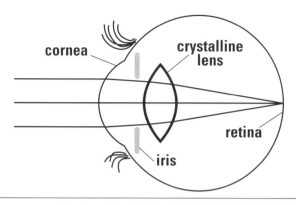

Figure 4 *The cornea and the crystalline lens both refract (bend) light, and both play an important role in focusing.*

Bending Light

In order to bring them to a focus, light rays must be bent (Figure 2). A *converging lens* brings light rays to a focus; a *diverging lens* causes them to spread (Figure 3). Both kinds of lenses are used to help people with vision problems.

This bending of light rays by a lens is called *refraction*. In the eye, light is bent first at the cornea, where it enters the eye, and then again at the crystalline lens (Figure 4). An eye that doesn't focus light properly is said to have a *refractive error*. The goal of laser vision correction is the reduction or elimination of refractive errors.

Because it aims to correct refractive errors, laser vision correction is a form of *refractive surgery*. All refractive surgery works by changing the eye very slightly so as to allow light to be refracted (bent) a little differently. These small changes let the eye focus light on the retina and give the patient clear vision.

In Chapter 4 we will look closely at the common refractive errors. Before we do that, however, it will help to look at how the normal eye works.

The Cornea

The cornea is the clear dome at the center of the eye through which we see. Because it is clear and lets light into the eye, the cornea is sometimes likened to a window.

The cornea is a remarkable structure: it and the crystalline lens are the only transparent organs that we have, and the cornea is the only structure that gets the oxygen it needs directly from the air instead of

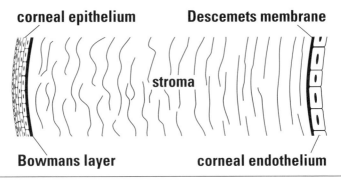

Figure 5 *The cornea is a five-layer structure. The topmost layer is the epithelium, a thin skim of cells that protects the cornea from the external environment. Below that is Bowmans layer, a thin layer that forms the border between the epithelium and the stroma. The stroma is a solid bed of transparent tissue that supports the cornea and represents 90% of corneal thickness. The stroma is the part of the cornea that is sculpted during laser vision correction. Below the stroma are two thin layers: Descemets membrane and the corneal endothelium.*

from the blood stream. (Blood vessels in the cornea would block our vision!) At night when the eyes are closed for sleep, the cornea gets dissolved oxygen from the tear film, which gets its oxygen from the tiny blood vessels on the inside of the eyelids.

Many people think that all of the eye's focusing is done by the crystalline lens. But that isn't the case. Fully two-thirds of the eye's focusing power comes from the cornea! This is an important fact for laser refractive surgery. Because the cornea plays a major role in refraction, a small reshaping of the cornea can change an eye that can't quite focus into an eye that focuses normally.

Although the cornea looks like a simple piece of clear tissue, it is a beautifully organized five-layer structure (Figure 5). The top layer, the *epithelium,* seals the cornea from the environment. Just a few cell layers thick, the epithelium repairs itself quickly if it is injured. (Some laser vision procedures require that the epithelium be removed. It grows back completely in just 3 or 4 days.)

Just below the epithelium is *Bowmans layer*, a thin layer that separates the epithelium from the *stroma*. The stroma is clear tissue that makes up most of the corneal thickness.

Beneath the stroma is another layer called *Descemets membrane*. And under Descemets membrane is a very important single layer of cells called the *endothelium*, which maintains the balance of water and nutrients in the cornea.

In refractive surgery, the most important layers are the epithelium and the stroma. We'll talk more about them in the sections on LASIK and PRK.

Behind the Cornea

Directly behind the cornea is the *iris*, which gives the eye its attractive color. The hole in the center of the iris which lets light into the eye is called the *pupil*. The iris reacts automatically to light, making the pupil smaller in bright light and enlarging the pupil in response to reduced light.

Just behind the iris is the crystalline lens. The crystalline lens can change shape to adjust the focussing power of the eye. This allows the eye to focus on near objects, like this book, as well as on distant ones. The process of changing focus from distance to near is called *accommodation*. Accommodation takes place so rapidly that we are usually unaware of it.

Most refractive surgery (and all laser vision correction) is done at the surface of the eye (the cornea) and doesn't affect the crystalline lens. For people with extreme near- or farsightedness, there are new procedures that involve the crystalline lens instead of the cornea. While they hold great promise, these procedures are limited to use in people with very strong refractive errors. We will talk about them in Chapter 8.

As we age, however, the crystalline lens slowly loses its ability to change shape. As this happens, we gradually lose our ability to accommodate. Although this process starts when we are very young, most people don't notice its effects until sometime around their 40th year. Then they begin to have difficulty reading when the light is poor (as in many restaurants) or when the type is small (like the phone

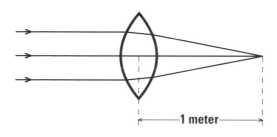

Figure 6 *A 1-diopter converging lens. By definition, a +1.00 D lens brings parallel rays of light to a focus 1 meter behind the lens.*

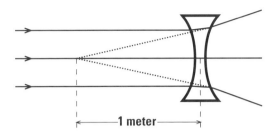

Figure 7 *A 1-diopter diverging lens (a −1.00 D lens) causes parallel rays to diverge. If one traces the rays backwards, one finds a "virtual focus" 1 meter in front of the lens.*

book). This is why, after age 45, most people need reading glasses.

Doctors call this gradual loss of accommodation *presbyopia*, which translates as "older eye." Presbyopia is entirely normal and happens to everyone, starting sometime around age 40. As we will see in later chapters, presbyopia has some implications for people considering refractive surgery.

The Retina

The retina is an extremely complex organ that "translates" the energy from light that enters the eye into nerve impulses that are sent to the brain. What is important for laser vision correction is that if the image that the cornea/crystalline lens optical system puts on the retina is out of focus, what we see will be blurred. The goal of laser vision correction is to gently reshape the cornea so that eye is able to put a focussed image on the retina.

The Power of the Eye

Anyone familiar with lenses knows that some lenses are more pow-

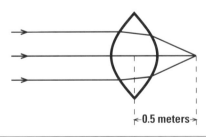

Figure 8 *A 2.00 D lens is twice as strong as a 1.00 D lens, which means that it can bring light to a focus in half the distance.*

erful than others. We measure lens power in a unit called *diopters*. (The symbol for diopters is the letter D.) If a lens causes light rays to converge, its power (in diopters) has a plus sign. A lens that causes rays of light to diverge has a minus sign before its power.

Let's look at some examples. A 1-diopter converging lens (a +1.00 D lens) is defined as a lens with the ability to bring parallel rays of light to a focus 1 meter behind the lens (Figure 6). A −1.00 D lens is equally powerful. It just causes light rays to diverge instead of converge (Figure 7).

A +2.00 D lens is twice as strong as +1.00 D lens, which means that the +2.00 D lens can focus light in half the distance required by a +1.00 D lens (Figure 8). If you look at the +1.00 and +2.00 lenses, you will notice that the stronger lens, the +2.00 D lens, is more steeply curved.

In the eye, the cornea and crystalline lens taken together are a +66.00 D optical system. This is a very powerful optical system, and it allows the normal eye to bring parallel light rays to a focus on the retina, which is less than an inch behind the cornea. An eye that has a refractive error, say an eye that is a little weak at +64.00 D, will see normally with +2.00 D glasses or contact lenses.

As we will see in the next section, it is easy to measure how nearsighted or how farsighted a person is. Later, when we explain laser vision correction, we will show how the excimer laser changes the shape of the cornea to give it additional plus or minus power. This small change in refractive power gives a farsighted, nearsighted, or even an astigmatic eye exactly the refracting system it needs!

Visual Acuity

One last topic needs to be covered before we go on to look at nearsightedness: how vision is measured. Most people are familiar with the term 20/20 and know that person who is 20/20 has normal vision. But what exactly does 20/20 mean?

The system for measuring visual acuity (sharpness) comes down to us from a 19th century German eye doctor named Snellen, who had noticed that the oil lamps on a carriage approaching his house appeared as a single dot of light when the carriage was far off. As the carriage approached, there came a point where he could tell there were actually two lamps. For people with good distance vision the point at which the single dot of light revealed itself as two separate lamps was farther off than for people with poor distance vision.

Snellen used this observation as the basis for creating the eye chart

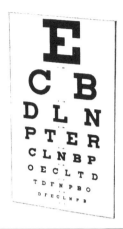

Figure 9 *A Snellen eye chart. Sometimes people talk about "gaining (or losing) a line of vision." A person who gains a line can read one more line on the eye chart than he could before. A person who has lost a line of vision is able to read one less line. (From Stein HA, Slatt BJ, Stein RM:* The Ophthalmic Assistant *ed 6. St. Louis, Mosby-Yearbook, 1994. Reprinted with permission.)*

we know today (Figure 9). Instead of asking patients to distinguish carriage lamps at dusk (a hopelessly impractical, albeit romantic, idea), he used letters. And instead of moving the chart to find the point at which the patient could make out the letters, Snellen used different sized letters and worked with the patient to find the smallest letters the patient could read.

The Snellen chart is read at a uniform distance of 20 feet (6 meters). A normal eye is defined as one that can just read a certain size type at 20 feet. A patient who has 20/20 vision can read at 20 feet the same line of type that the person with normal vision can read at 20 feet. At 20 feet away, the patient who is a little bit nearsighted might only be able to read the line that a normal eye could read at 40 feet. This nearsighted person is said to have 20/40 vision. Similarly, if the best a patient can do at 20 feet is read what a normal eye can see at 200 feet, the patient is said to have 20/200 vision.

Is it possible to have better than 20/20 vision? Yes. A person with really sharp vision who can read a line at 20 feet that the normal eye can read only at 15 feet is said to have 20/15 vision.

The 20/20 notation is a measure of *visual acuity*, which is sometimes called "Snellen acuity." A good benchmark is that while 20/20 is considered good normal vision, most states and provinces issue driver's licenses to people with 20/40 vision or better.

How Strong is Your Correction?

If you are nearsighted, farsighted, or have astigmatism, you probably wear either glasses or contact lenses. For reasons that we will go into in the next chapter, if you are nearsighted, your glasses or contacts will act as a diverging lens. People who are farsighted need correction by means of a converging lens.

If you are just a little bit nearsighted, you can use a low-power lens, perhaps –2.00 D. If you are moderately nearsighted, you will require a stronger correction, say –4.50 D. If you are very nearsighted, you might require correction of –10.00 D or more.

There are two common ways to describe the quality of your vision. One way is to use Snellen acuity and say the individual has, for example, 20/200 vision. Another way is ask: How much correction is necessary for the eye to see 20/20? If you are nearsighted and –3.25 D corrects you to 20/20, then you are said to be –3.25 D, meaning that –3.25 D is what is needed to get your best vision. (It's possible, of course, that you have a different correction in each eye. If that were the case, we might say, for example, that you were –3.25 D in your left eye and –4.50 D in your right eye.)

As we shall see in subsequent chapters, the amount of correction you need, and whether it requires a diverging (minus) or converging (plus) lens for correction, will play a role in determining your laser vision correction.

CHAPTER 4

Errors of Refraction

Introduction

Nearsightedness, farsightedness, and *astigmatism* are common vision problems that affect millions of people. We refer to them as *refractive errors* because they all result from the eye's inability to bend (refract) light so as to focus it precisely on the retina.

Until recently, people with refractive errors could see clearly only by wearing corrective glasses or contact lenses. Today, all that has been changed by laser vision correction. Now people with refractive errors have options that didn't exist as recently as 10 years ago.

In this chapter we will explore what it means to be nearsighted, farsighted, or to have astigmatism. Understanding these refractive errors is a necessary foundation for understanding how laser vision correction can make it possible to see clearly without correction.

Nearsightedness/Myopia

The medical name for nearsightedness is *myopia*, and doctors refer to a nearsighted person as a *myope*. In Chapter 3 we saw that, in an eye that focuses normally (called an *emmetropic* eye), the cornea and crystalline lens work together to bring rays of light to a focus on the retina (Figure 1).

In myopia, the cornea/lens optical system is, in effect, too strong for the eye. The result is that light comes to a focus in front of the retina, and the image on the retina is slightly out of focus (Figure 2). Sometimes, eye doctors will say that a myopic eye is "too long," meaning that it is too long for the power of the cornea/crystalline lens optical system.

Myopia is called nearsightedness because, without correction, myopes can see an object clearly only if it is close. ("Close" means a few feet to a few inches, depending the degree of myopia.) Myopes can see distant objects clearly with the help of a *diverging lens*. Using a diverging lens—in the form of glasses or contact lenses—will move the focal point back

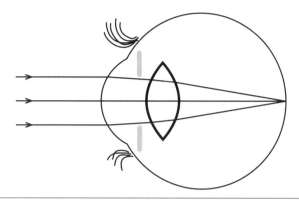

Figure 1 *In the emmetropic (normal) eye, the cornea/crystalline lens optical system brings light rays to a focus on the retina.*

to the retina. (Figure 3). The goal of laser vision correction for myopia is to modify the shape of the cornea so that light passing through it from a distant object will come to a focus on the retina.

Farsightedness/Hyperopia

Farsighted individuals have a condition called *hyperopia*; eye doctors call someone with hyperopia a *hyperope*. Hyperopia is just the opposite of myopia: in hyperopia, the cornea/lens optical system is too weak, so light entering they eye comes to focus a behind the retina. For this reason, hyperopes are said to have eyes that are "too short." (Figure 4). Hyperopes tend to be able to see distant objects clearly, but they can't focus clearly on things nearby.

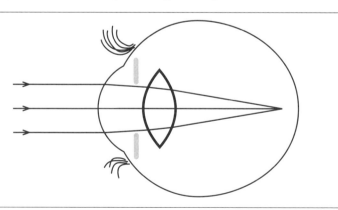

Figure 2 *In the myopic (nearsighted) eye, light comes to a focus in front of the retina. This eye's optical is system is too strong; The eye is said to be "too long" (for its optical system).*

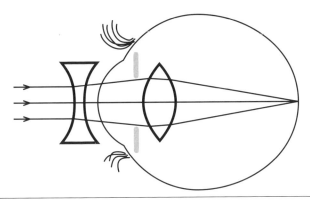

Figure 3 *A diverging lens in front of the eye moves the myope's focus back to the retina.*

Of course, the idea of a focal point behind the retina is purely theoretical. Light doesn't get through the retina. Instead, it lands on the retina slightly out of focus. As a result, the image seen is blurred. Hyperopes can get the additional refractive power they need by using a converging (plus power) lens (Figure 5).

Astigmatism

Astigmatism is a relatively simple problem. Describing it, however, is made difficult by the fact that astigmatism has to be understood in three dimensions, and it is very difficult to show three dimensions on a two-dimensional piece of paper!

Astigmatism occurs when the cornea or the crystalline lens (usu-

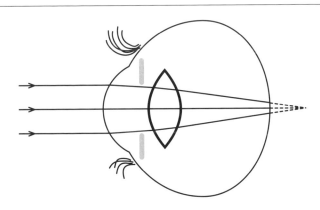

Figure 4 *The hyperope's optical system is too weak. The focal point is behind the retina. The eye is said to be "too short."*

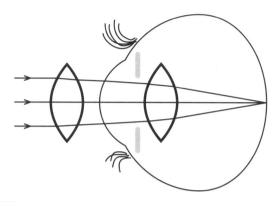

Figure 5 *A converging lens gives the hyperope the extra power needed to bring light to a focus on the retina.*

ally the cornea) has different curvatures in different meridians. (A meridian is a line that goes around the surface of a sphere. For example, the Equator is a meridian on the earth. Similarly any straight line drawn along the surface of the globe that connects the North Pole to the South Pole would be a meridian.) When the cornea has a different curvature in different meridians, it will have different optical powers in each meridian. And when this happens, there is no single point on which light entering the eye can focus. Instead, the focus is spread out.

One way to conceptualize astigmatism is by comparing the shape of a softball to the shape of a football. The softball is a perfect sphere. If you had a glass softball and cut off the front one-third to make a lens out of it, the front surface would be a piece of a sphere (Figure 6). Every meridian

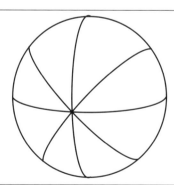

Figure 6 *Meridians drawn on the surface of a piece of a sphere. Because this is spherical, each meridian has exactly the same curvature.*

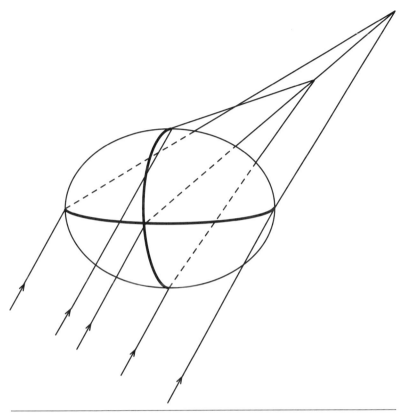

Figure 7 *A "football-shaped" lens with meridians drawn. Note that the meridian drawn over the long axis will be flatter than the meridian drawn on the short axis. You can see also that the lens is more powerful at the steeper short axis, where it brings light to a focus in less distance than is required at the flatter long axis.*

on your "softball lens" would have the same curvature.

Now take a glass football and do the same thing. The lens has a different shape. On the short axis of the football, the lens is steeper and has more power. On the long axis, the lens is less steep and has less power. This lens can't bring light to a single focus (Figure 7). The "football lens" is like an astigmatic eye: different curvatures in different meridians make it impossible for the lens to bring light to a single focus.

The amount of astigmatism is the difference (in diopters) between the most powerful meridian and the least powerful meridian. If that difference is 2.00 diopters, then they eye is said to have 2.00 D of astigmatism. The greater the difference in power between the meridians, the higher the astigmatism; and the higher the astigmatism, the worse the vision. Small amounts of astigmatism are very common, and most myopes have at least some astigmatism. About one-third of myopes have 1.00 D or more of astigmatism.

How Much Refractive Error?

Refractive error is measured in diopters. When your eyes are measured for glasses, the eye doctor or technician uses a device called a *phoropter* to put a series of trial lenses in front of your eyes. The person measuring your refractive error keeps testing until he or she finds the lens that gives you the best vision you can achieve. This process of trying lenses is called a *refraction*. At the end of the refraction, you are usually given a slip of paper with your prescription.

The prescription is simply the power of the spectacle lens that will correct your refractive error. A nearsighted eye that is 3.00 D too strong, for example, will get a prescription for a –3.00 D lens. (This can be made up in either glasses or contact lenses.) Myopes, whose eyes are too strong, always have minus power corrections. By the same token, an eye that is too weak (that is, a hyperopic eye) needs a plus power lens.

Presbyopia

We discussed presbyopia in the last chapter because it is a perfectly normal part of growing older. The underlying problem in presbyopia is a crystalline lens that can no longer change shape to accommodate. As a result, laser vision correction, which works on the cornea at the surface of the eye, can't deal with the root cause of presbyopia. Nonetheless, there are some things that can be done with laser vision correction to help the presbyope.

For most people, becoming presbyopic means losing the ability to read without glasses (or some other correction). The exception is people with small amounts of myopia. Even when they become presbyopic, they can often read without glasses. A little bit of myopia is not entirely bad! Of course, the older myope who can read without glasses will not have sharp distance vision.

Once presbyopia sets in, an eye needs a different correction for distance vision and for near. Thus, presbyopes must wear glasses with bifocal, trifocal, or "no-line" (progressive) lenses.

Monovision

One solution for presbyopes is called *monovision*. This has also

"I'm looking forward to going sailing."

NAME: Virginia Gibberd
AGE: 42
OCCUPATION: Business Manager, CTV Sports
PROCEDURE: LASIK for high myopia and astigmatism
OPHTHALMOLOGIST: Dr. Albert Cheskes
BEFORE LASER VISION CORRECTION: Unable to count fingers more than four feet distant*
AFTER LASER VISION CORRECTION: 20/20

Before undergoing treatment, Virginia talked with a colleague—the head of health reporting at CTV in Toronto.

She's in news, and they have to show both sides of every issue. She had heard great things about laser vision correction, and she wanted to know, realistically, if there were problems. And she couldn't find any. That to me was a really good sign. There had been no negative reports. She put ads in the paper twice, looking for people with bad results, and she couldn't find anyone who had had anything go wrong.

Virginia had a consultation at the Bochner Eye Institute with Dr. Cheskes on a Tuesday and then scheduled an appointment for LASIK surgery on the following Saturday.

I'm a quick decision-maker. I do it for a living. To me laser vision correction just made absolute sense.

I describe it to people, and they go 'oooh!' They don't like the thought of anything in their eye. But the recovery time is quick. I was astounded by that, and I was astounded

---

Before laser vision correction, Virginia's uncorrected vision was too impaired to measure using conventional scales.

that I walked out within 30 minutes. You sit there for 20 minutes, then they look at your eye and say, 'Oh ah that looks great,' and then bye! Off you go. It's quite phenomenal.

I woke up the day after the first eye was done and I told my husband what time it was. Before, I couldn't read the clock from the other side of the room. But the morning after the procedure, even wearing the little eye shield, I was able to read it. Usually I would be holding my watch an inch from my eye. It was pretty phenomenal to realize it was such a drastic change. I was playing golf a couple days after the second eye.

The best thing is having clarity of sight all the time. When you have myopia like I had, you really are handicapped. Now, I'm looking forward to going sailing. I'm also looking forward to going swimming underwater and being able to open my eyes and see.

been labeled omnivision because it enables the individual to see all areas, far and near. In monovision, one eye is corrected for distance and the other eye for near. This is often done with contact lenses. For example, a patient who was emmetropic—that is, who didn't need correction for distance—could be a given a near-vision contact lens to wear in one eye. That way, she could see distance clearly with the uncorrected eye and see up close with the contact lens eye.

The good news about monovision is that it works pretty well in most people. Monovision isn't for everybody, however. Between 20% and 30% of patients who try monovision have trouble getting used to it. These patients prefer bifocal correction and usually return to it.

The downside to monovision is that it reduces the quality of vision. It just makes sense that you can see better at distance using two eyes than you can with just one eye. The same is true of near vision. You can use two eyes to see both distance and near with bifocal glasses. Of course, the downside to bifocal glasses is that you have to wear glasses! The bottom line with presbyopia is that *any* form of vision correction, including laser vision correction, requires some sort of compromise. And presbyopia happens to everyone—there are no exceptions!

Presbyopia and Laser Vision Correction

What does presbyopia mean for laser vision correction? If a 45 year old myope who is used to reading without glasses gets laser vision correction that gives him 20/20 vision at distance, he suddenly won't be able to read without glasses. An easy solution is reading glasses.

Another solution is monovision. Just as with contact lenses, laser vision correction can leave one eye set for distance and the other eye corrected for reading. This solution works well for many people; but the only way to know if it will work for you is to try it in advance with contact lenses. Disposable contact lens make this easy and fun to try.

Let's go back for a moment to the 45-year-old myope whose laser vision correction suddenly caused him to need glasses for reading. It is important to realize that his problem was his presbyopia not his surgery! A completely normal person who has had 20/20 distance vision for her entire life will need help reading at some point in her 40s. People 45 and older who are 20/20 for distance don't have the ability to see clearly up close without correction.

If you are under 40, the chances are that monovision won't be of much interest to you now. However, we think it's worth knowing about monovision, because there is a time in everyone's life when presbyopia becomes a problem. At that point, it is worth knowing that laser vision correction may allow you to correct one eye for reading.

CHAPTER 5

Creating New Eyes: How Laser Vision Correction Works

Introduction

From the patient's perspective, laser vision correction is a relatively quick and easy procedure. It's over in a few minutes, and the ophthalmologist and the laser do most of the work. The laser, however, is one of those simple-seeming inventions whose ease of use hides its underlying technological wizardry. It's like the telephone. The telephone is easy to use—just push a few buttons and you're connected to the house next door. Push the buttons differently and you are talking to a friend in Rio de Janeiro; push the buttons yet again and you're on the line with a business associate in Tokyo. When you think about it, it's quite a miracle.

The excimer laser has some of the same miracle quality. A few minutes or seconds under the laser, a very brief healing period, and suddenly you can see much better than before! To many who experience it, it feels exactly like a miracle.

As with every important invention, creating the excimer laser took enormous creativity—indeed, it took true genius. First came the all-important realization that the excimer laser could reshape corneal tissue and thereby help eyes with refractive errors focus properly. Once it was realized that the excimer laser *could* reshape the cornea, there came years of dogged engineering studies and clinical testing that slowly turned the excimer laser into an instrument of breathtaking precision. We'll see how it works in this chapter.

The excimer laser's extraordinary precision is the key to its ability to reshape corneal tissue. How precise is the excimer laser? It is so precise that it can produce changes in refraction that are too small for us to measure in a standard refraction.

How the Laser Works

The laser used to re-shape corneal tissue is called an *excimer laser* (Figure 1). The excimer laser uses tiny amounts of two gases, argon and fluorine, to produce a beam of a single wavelength (193 nanometers) of ultraviolet light. This light is actually invisible to us—people can't see ultraviolet—but we can see its effects. The beam from the excimer is focused with extreme accuracy.

One of the reasons that the excimer laser works so well for vision correction is that all of the energy from the beam is absorbed right at the surface of the eye, where the beam strikes. (This is a function of the wavelength. Visible light can penetrate the cornea; but light at the 193-nanometer wavelength is absorbed at the corneal surface, and does not penetrate deeply. This makes the laser safe for use on eyes.) Because light at this wavelength is absorbed right at the surface, the excimer beam removes corneal tissue a few molecular layers at a time, and only at the very surface.

How does the laser remove tissue? Energy from the beam breaks up the molecules it strikes and vaporizes them, without damaging the surrounding tissue. This ultraprecise vaporization of tiny amounts of tissue is called *ablation*.

The ophthalmologist doing the laser vision correction procedure can control the laser with great precision. He can control exactly how

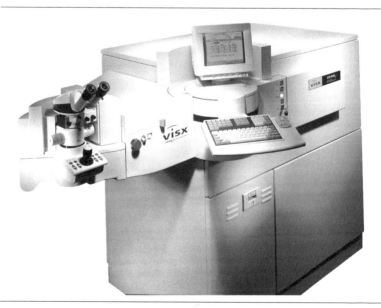

Figure 1 *An excimer laser. (Photo courtesy of VISX, Incorporated.)*

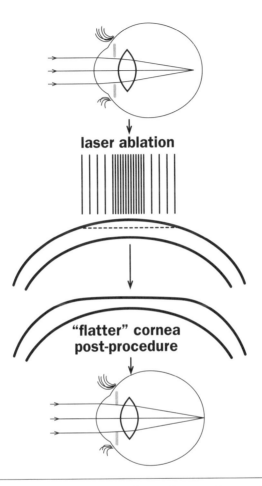

Figure 2 *Top In the myopic (nearsighted) eye, the optical system is too strong. Light is bent to a focus in front of the retina.* **Middle** *Ablation removes a small amount of tissue from the central cornea.* **Bottom** *The flatter cornea acts as a weaker lens. Now the eye is able to focus light on the retina.*

much energy is focussed on the eye and determine the pattern in which the laser "deposits" energy on the cornea. By controlling these two elements, he can determine the exact amount of tissue to be ablated and the shape of the ablated area.

Correcting Refraction

We have said that a myopic eye is "too strong." By that we meant that the myope's cornea/lens optical system bends light too much and brings it to a focus in front of the retina (Figure 2). By ablating the

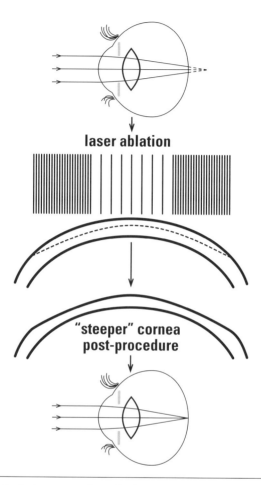

laser ablation

**"steeper" cornea
post-procedure**

Figure 3 *Top In the hyperopic (farsighted) eye, the optical system is too weak to bring light to a focus on the retina.* **Middle** *Ablation removes more tissue from the peripheral cornea than the center, creating a steeper cornea.* **Bottom** *The new corneal shape acts as a stronger lens. Now the eye is able to bring light to a focus on the retina.*

central portion of the cornea, we lessen the steepness of the curve, and thereby lower the power of the cornea. (Ophthalmologists describe this as "flattening" the cornea slightly.) After ablation, the eye is able to bring light from distant objects to a focus on the retina.

The opposite happens with hyperopia. In hyperopia, we need to steepen the cornea to make the optical system stronger (Figure 3). This is done by ablating tissue from the periphery of the cornea, in effect steepening the cornea and giving it added refractive power.

Astigmatism is handled in a similar fashion. In astigmatism, the same cornea has a steeper and a flatter axis. To correct this, more tissue is removed from the steeper axis, reducing its optical power and making the surface of the cornea more like a part of a sphere.

How much tissue is ablated to get this refractive correction? In myopia, it's possible to get a significant refractive correction by removing a layer of tissue just 50 microns thick. How thick is 50 microns? A micron is 1/1000th of a millimeter. How thick is that? A credit card is about 1 millimeter thick. So a 50 micron layer of tissue is about 5% of the thickness of a credit card. That is roughly the thickness of a human hair. It is awesome to think that all that may stand between you and good natural vision is a hairsbreadth of corneal tissue!

The Actual Operations

So far, we have discussed the theory. Now, how does laser vision correction work in practice? There are two ways in which the laser can be used to ablate tissue and provide a refractive correction. One technique is called PRK, for photorefractive keratectomy. (This translates as: [*photo*] using light; [*refractive*] to get a refractive change; [*kera*] by corneal; [*ectomy*] tissue removal.) Photorefractive keratectomy is hard to say, and so doctors, patients, staff, and laypeople use the initials, PRK. PRK was the first successful form of laser vision correction, and it is still in widespread use.

The other common technique is a little newer. It's called LASIK, for laser in situ keratomileusis. As with PRK, no one (not even a doctor) uses the term "laser in situ keratomileusis." Instead, everyone says LASIK (pronounced *lay'zick*).

PRK

PRK works on the very surface of the cornea. In PRK there are two important steps: (1) removal of the corneal epithelium, followed by (2) the ablation of the stroma that lies just below the epithelium. (It may help to refer back to Chapter 3 to review the structure of the cornea.)

In order to ablate the stroma (which is necessary for the refractive correction), it is first necessary to remove the epithelium. This can be done in a variety of ways. Some ophthalmologists use the laser itself to remove the epithelium; others use alcohol, or a brush, or a simple hand-held instrument that is designed for epithelium removal. All told, removal of the epithelium should take no more than 1–2 minutes, and is painless.

Once the epithelium has been removed, the ophthalmologist uses the laser, which he has already programmed with the patient's refractive correction, to ablate the stroma in a precise pattern that will produce the desired change in refraction. After less than a minute under the laser, the operation is over.

Because the epithelium, the thin protective cover of the cornea, has been removed, right after PRK the patient is given a bandage contact lens that will shield the cornea during the 3 or 4 days it takes for new epithelial cells to grow. After the epithelium regrows, the eye heals slowly over a period of weeks (or months) until the final visual result is obtained. However, the most rapid healing takes place in the first few weeks after PRK. In the remaining time, the eye slowly stabilizes at its final correction. Usually, PRK patients can go back to work and resume a normal life 3 days after their procedure.

LASIK

The refractive ablation performed in LASIK is almost identical to the ablation in PRK. In LASIK, however, the epithelium is not removed. Instead, the ophthalmologist gets to the stroma by using a device called a microkeratome to cut a thin flap of corneal tissue. This flap is curled back to reveal a bed of stroma beneath (Figure 4).

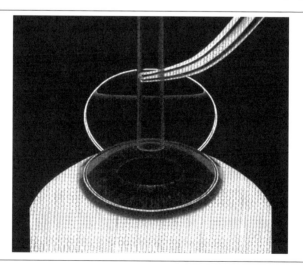

Figure 4 *After the microkeratome has cut a thin flap of corneal tissue, the flap is turned back like the page of a book to reveal the stroma. (From Stein HA, Cheskes AT, Stein RM:* The Excimer: Fundamentals and Clinical Use. *Thorofare, NJ, Slack, Incorporated, 1997. Reprinted with permission.)*

The laser then works, reshaping the stromal bed. After the laser is finished (a matter of perhaps a minute), the flap is repositioned over the stroma.

The repositioned flap fits tightly, and there is no need for stitches to hold it in place. Even in the very rare instance where a flap is cut off completely—called a "free cap"—there is no problem. After the ablation, the cap is simply placed back on the eye, and the eye heals as it would in a typical LASIK. (Just like with a flap, natural suction holds the cap in place.)

Because the corneal epithelium has been kept intact, there is no need for a bandage contact lens following LASIK. In addition, there is less pain associated with LASIK. And visual recovery is more rapid after LASIK than PRK. The downside to LASIK is that it is a more complex procedure (so it takes a little longer), and there is the added risk of problems due to the flap. In the end, however, the visual results of PRK and LASIK are very similar. Both procedures can produce excellent results.

CHAPTER 6

The Experience of PRK

Introduction

People often want to know what it feels like to have laser vision correction. In this chapter, we will walk you through the entire PRK procedure. We will try to recreate the experience from the moment you come to the laser center until you leave. We'll also cover the post-procedure recovery period. Our aim is to give you an idea of what it would feel like to have PRK. If you eventually do have PRK, this should help prepare you for the experience.

Like so many things in life, worrying about PRK is much worse than the actual procedure. The reality is that PRK is quick and virtually painless. (There may, however, be minimal discomfort in the 3–4 days following PRK.) The bottom line is: there is far less to worry about in the reality of PRK (or LASIK) than a person unfamiliar with the procedure might imagine.

As we walk you through the day of the procedure, we will use our institution, the Bochner Eye Institute in downtown Toronto, as an example. Are the steps we go through radically different from what happens at other centers? No. To stay abreast of the state of the art in laser vision correction, we visit centers around the world; and eye doctors from around the world come to the Bochner Eye Institute. We do this to learn from one another. So we know that the steps that you go through at the Bochner Eye Institute are similar to what you experience at any world class laser vision correction center.

What's the difference between our center and others? It's in the details. It's in our attention to your needs. It's in our willingness to listen to you. It's in the experience of our physicians and their dedication to excellence in the care of your vision.

Contact Lens Wear

Many of the people who have laser vision correction are former contact lens wearers. It is very important that, at the time of laser vision correction, your corneas be free of the effects of contact lens wear. (Wearing contact lenses, particularly rigid lenses, can subtly affect the shape of the cornea. When contact lens wear stops, the cornea goes back to its natural shape over a period of days or weeks.) Your eye doctor will tell you precisely how far in advance you must stop lens wear, but at the Bochner Eye Institute, we have the following general rules:

- No soft contact lens wear for 2–3 days prior to laser vision correction.
- No gas permeable or hard lens wear for 2–3 weeks prior to laser vision correction. (For an individual who has worn rigid lenses for more than 10 years, an even longer lens-free period may be required.)

Before You Come In

As the day of the procedure draws near, you can expect to feel a mix of eager excitement tempered by a bit of nervous tension. This is entirely normal. Almost everybody comes to the procedure with a lot of anticipation and a touch of worry.

Happily, there are few restrictions to worry about on the day of your laser vision correction procedure. You can eat and drink whatever you wish (except alcohol). If you are on medications, you can continue to take them as you normally would. (Be sure, however, that your eye doctor knows about those medications before the day of the procedure!) Women coming in for laser vision correction should not wear eye makeup.

Most people dress casually and comfortably for their procedure. (You'll remain in your street clothes during the procedure.) You may want to have a friend come with you to the center for companionship. In many centers, ours included, the companion can stay with you every step of the way. If getting to the center requires driving, you'll need someone to drive you on the way home.

One small piece of instruction: on the day of your procedure, it's important to avoid alcohol or any kind of drug that is likely to leave you feeling drowsy. During the procedure, you'll be asked to keep your gaze fixed on a red blinking light. This helps position the laser on the center of your cornea. It is much easier to maintain fixation for the few minutes of the procedure if you are fully alert.

Arriving at the Center

At the Bochner Eye Institute, a member of the staff will greet you on arrival, and if you haven't been there before, show you the facility. We do this to help you feel comfortable and familiarize you with the

"I've recommended PRK to 40 or 50 other people."

NAME: Loreen Rudd
AGE: 37
OCCUPATION: Homemaker, small business owner, volunteer
PROCEDURE: PRK for myopia and astigmatism
OPHTHALMOLOGIST: Dr. Harold Stein
BEFORE LASER VISION CORRECTION: 20/400
AFTER LASER VISION CORRECTION: 20/20

Before the PRK procedure, I wasn't blind when I wasn't wearing glasses or contacts, but my distance vision was very blurry, and I had a hard time making out specific images. I wasn't able to find my way around when I woke up, and I would bump into things constantly. I always had bruises on my legs.

I decided that the risk of PRK was minimal. I knew three people who had had it done, and I'd looked at it extensively. There is a very small risk, but I figured you're also taking a risk when you put a contact lens in your eye, since that can damage the cornea.

One of the interesting things about the procedure is that you think you're going to see the doctor's hand—all you actually see through the whole thing is this little red dot they ask you to stare at. By the time you want it to be over, and you're getting nervous, it's over!

I have a very good idea of how much my vision has improved. When I was 7 years old, I used to play games with my brother of 'how far can you see.' I noticed as my vision gradually deteriorated, and I remember what I was able to see without correction before I used glasses or contacts. Since the PRK procedure, I can see as well as I did when I was 7 years old.

Now, my vision is so good I keep thinking that I must have contacts in my eyes. I take my new vision for granted. I don't have to wash my glasses anymore, and I can just go out without worrying about my glasses getting steamed-up inside the car. I've recommended PRK to 40 or 50 other people. It's something I totally stand behind.

surroundings. Sometimes, seeing the facility will bring up a question that we will be happy to answer for you. Any final tests or measurements that need to be completed prior to your procedure will be handled shortly after you arrive.

Before the procedure takes place, your ophthalmologist and members of the Bochner Eye Institute staff will review the procedure with you and answer any final questions you may have. If you have *any* concerns, or if there's anything more you feel you might like to know, this is the time to ask. Your questions and concerns are very important. The procedure will go better for everyone—even the doctor—if you come to it without nagging questions or worries.

Medications
About one-half hour before your procedure you will start to get eye drops. There will be three kinds of drops:
- *Anesthetic* drops will numb the eye and make the procedure painless.
- *Antibiotic* eye drops are given to prevent infection.
- *Anti-inflammatory* drops will help reduce discomfort and speed recovery after the procedure.

Preparing for the Procedure
After the eye drops have been given, you (and the person accompanying you) will be taken to the room where the laser is located. At this point, the laser is already programmed with your correction. The

chair in which you will lie back for the procedure will be adjusted for you, and the eye that isn't being treated will be covered.

After you are comfortable, your ophthalmologist will greet you again and put an eyelid holder in place to keep you from blinking. As he proceeds, your ophthalmologist will talk to you, explaining what he is doing at each step. As the procedure continues, he will let you know what to expect next.

Removing the Epithelium

The first step in the PRK procedure is to remove the epithelium. This can be done in a number of ways. Some ophthalmologists use the laser to do it. Others use a special instrument to simply wipe the epithelium away. Still other doctors use alcohol or a brush-like device. All of these methods work well. The choice of technique depends on your ophthalmologist's preference and on specific factors related to your eye. However it is done, removing the epithelium is painless and is over in less than 2 minutes.

The Laser

Next the laser is put in position, and you will be asked to fix your gaze on a blinking red light. (As the procedure progresses, it may become more difficult to see the light. This is entirely normal.) Then the ophthalmologist activates the laser and the procedure begins.

While the laser is operating, you will be asked to keep your head still and your eye fixed on the light. You should try your best, but you don't have to be absolutely perfect at this. A small amount of eye movement won't affect the outcome. In addition, the ophthalmologist will be watching closely. If there is too much movement, he will stop the laser. You will then have a moment to relax before being asked if you are ready to start again. If you are ready, you will re-fix your gaze on the light, and the procedure will start back up. Patients often have to stop and re-fix their gaze. It is nothing to be concerned about.

Actual laser time for the whole procedure is usually around a minute per eye. During this time, you will experience the distinctive sounds and smells that are characteristic of the laser in operation. The laser makes a clicking sound when it operates. In addition, in the process of ablation, the laser vaporizes a tiny amount of tissue, which it is often possible to smell. Patients often describe this as an odd, somewhat unpleasant odor. Like the clicking sound, this is perfectly normal and to be expected.

When It's Over

When the treatment ends, the ophthalmologist will insert a "bandage" soft contact lens and then remove the eyelid holder. This thin, flexible lens will protect your eye during the 3 or 4 days that it takes the epithelium to regrow.

If you are having both eyes done (which is typically the case these days), it will take just a few moments to prepare the second eye for treatment. Then the process will be repeated. Your total time in the laser room will probably be under 20 minutes. (If you are having only one eye done, you will likely be out in 10 minutes.)

Leaving the Center

When the procedure is complete, additional antibiotic, anti-inflammatory, and analgesic (pain relieving) drops will be put in your eyes. The bandage lenses will remain in your eyes for the few (3–4) days it takes the epithelium to regrow. The bandage contact lens(es) should stay in your eye(s) for the entire time. Do not remove a lens unless told to do so by your eye doctor. Should a lens come out accidentally, contact your eye doctor right away.

When you leave the Bochner Eye Institute, we will give you a kit containing your medications and a schedule for taking them. It's important to take the eyedrops as you have been instructed.

Later that Day

It's a good idea to rest for the remainder of the day of your procedure. Anywhere from 30 to 90 minutes after the procedure, you may begin to feel some discomfort, as the drops that numbed your eyes for the procedure wear off.

At this point, people's responses vary. Some experience no pain at all. (It's not uncommon for a patient to say "I never felt a thing.") But other patients report mild to moderate pain. The people who experience this discomfort compare it to having a grain of sand in the eye. Some patients also report a slight burning sensation when they put in their eyedrops.

Rarely is the post-PRK pain serious, and it goes away entirely within a few days. If the discomfort bothers you, there is medication you can take. You can lessen the discomfort in the period right after the procedure by placing an icepack over your eyes and resting in a darkened room.

The Next Few Days

Some people experience a runny nose for a day or two following

An Optometrist's Approval

NAME: Dr. Cheryl Vincent, O.D.
OCCUPATION: Optometrist, co-owner,
VisionCare Associates,
East Lansing, MI
PROCEDURE: PRK for myopia
OPHTHALMOLOGIST: Dr. Raymond Stein
BEFORE LASER VISION CORRECTION: 20/400
AFTER LASER VISION CORRECTION: Better than 20/20

I've been in practice as an optometrist since 1986. I researched laser vision correction very thoroughly before I had the procedure done on my own eyes. Not only did I interview patients before and after they had laser vision correction, I also looked at their eyes myself. I examined people before the procedure and right after. I also looked at the eyes of people who had had laser vision correction years, months, and a few days earlier. In addition to that, I checked out the success rates of surgeons who specialize in laser vision correction. I wanted to know the number of patients they'd seen, and I was especially interested in their long-term success rates. All this research indicated to me that laser vision was safe, reliable, and effective. I scheduled an appointment with Dr. Raymond Stein.

Despite my knowledge of the procedure, I was still a bit nervous the morning I was to have it done. The doctors and staff put me at ease right away, however. They were professional and thorough. During the procedure I was completely relaxed. I was astonished at the speed of the procedure. The laser was operating on each eye for only 30 seconds! I had planned to have each eye done during a separate session, but almost immediately after having the first eye done, I could already see. And since the procedure was so easy, I asked them to do the second eye right then and there.

The change in my ability to see was immediate and dramatic. The day I had the procedure done, I was able to do simple things I hadn't done for 19 years, like watch television and see my face when it was more than a foot away from the mirror— *without glasses.* The day after surgery, I put my new, uncorrected vision to work, and went sightseeing in Toronto. I was able to drive a car just two days after the procedure.

One month after I returned home, my vision was better than 20/20. Trained optometrists and ophthalmologists need a microscope to see any irregularities in my corneas, and I have to tell them beforehand that I've had PRK, or they wouldn't know.

━━ • ━━

the procedure; and most patients report sensitivity to light in the period before the epithelium is completely healed (3–4 days after surgery).

Vision will be blurry until the epithelium heals, and you can expect to find it somewhat difficult to read for a few days immediately after the procedure. When the bandage contact lens is removed, close objects (say 6–10 feet) will look as if they are being seen through glasses coated with Vaseline. This condition will disappear as the surface of the eye heals to its original smoothness, generally within 1–2 weeks. You should be able to return to normal activity (including work) within 3 days after your procedure.

Your vision will become less blurry once the contact lens is removed. This should happen fairly quickly—most likely within a day or two. As the days go on and your vision improves even more, you may notice that your vision is a bit better on some days than on others. This fluctuating vision is rarely a significant problem; it should clear up completely on its own somewhere between 6 weeks and 6 months after the procedure.

Some people experience glare at night in the period following their procedure. (This is most pronounced in people who were high myopes prior to their procedure.) Night glare usually resolves slowly over time.

It's worth noting that the healing process is highly individual. Some people heal quickly after PRK; others heal more slowly. In most cases, patients are able to cope quite well, even though their eyes are still healing.

Follow-up

Follow-up is a very important part of PRK! Even if you think you're fine (and you are probably right), it's important to come in for scheduled checkups. There are two stages to the follow-up process. Immediately after your laser vision correction, you will have to come in for a quick appointment on each of the next three days after the procedure. At this appointment your eyes will be checked to see that they are healing properly and to be sure that there is no evidence of infection. On the third day, the bandage contact lens will be removed, if the epithelium is sufficiently healed.

In the next recovery stage, you will make brief follow-up visits in order to check on the healing process and measure the improvement in your vision. These visits will take place at 2 weeks, 1 month, and later dates on the direction of the managing eye doctor.

Restrictions

While people can get back to their normal activities quite soon after PRK, there are some important restrictions that you should heed during the recovery period:

- Do not expect to be able to drive for at least 3–5 days after the procedure. Thereafter, take it one day a time in deciding whether your vision has cleared sufficiently for you to drive safely.
- For the first week, do not swim or use hot tubs or whirlpools. It's OK to shower or bathe, but try to keep water and shampoo out of your eyes for the first few days.
- Avoid strenuous exercise for the first 2 days after the procedure so as not to dislodge the protective contact lenses. Rest as much as possible.
- During the first week avoid activities where you could get dust or other matter in your eyes. Things like gardening, wearing eye makeup, and dusty environments should be avoided.
- You will probably feel strain and irritation if you try to read or watch television for long periods during the first few days after

your procedure. Plan to take it easy for a few days. You will be fine soon enough!

● Smoking won't injure your eyes, but you may find that smoke is irritating for two to three days after PRK.

Your Vision

That's it! There's nothing more to PRK. If it seems like a fairly easy procedure, it should. It's a quick procedure with a relatively uneventful recovery period that is usually marked by steadily improving vision. By one month, your vision should be very close to its final correction; and by 3 months you should be getting used to your new life with good, *uncorrected* vision! Healing continues for at least 6 months, and as long as a year, but unlike the first week or two after surgery, you will no longer notice a change in your vision from day to day.

Because everyone heals differently, a small percentage of patients will want to have a second procedure to fine-tune vision in one or both eyes. This is called "enhancement." Patients at the Bochner Eye Institute are offered a lifetime enhancement policy that allows them to come in for additional "touch-up" procedures (at no cost) any time they wish!

CHAPTER 7

If You Have LASIK

Introduction

From the standpoint of correcting your vision, LASIK and PRK work in almost the same way. Both work by using a laser ablation to slightly alter the shape of the corneal stroma. The difference between LASIK and PRK is that in PRK the laser ablation is on the very surface of the eye, whereas in LASIK a surface flap is created, so that the laser can work just below the surface. The flap is then placed back over the ablated area.

In PRK, the ophthalmologist gets to the stroma by simply removing the epithelium and exposing the stroma. In LASIK, the ophthalmologist uses a device called a *microkeratome* (Figure 1) that produces a very thin flap of tissue from the surface of the cornea (Figure 2). This flap is turned back like the page of a book, allowing the laser to work in the exposed stromal bed. When the ablation is done, often in a minute or less, the flap is put back in place, and the procedure is over.

The advantage of LASIK is that it leaves the epithelium largely intact. The eye keeps its smooth refracting surface. (After PRK, it takes time for a smooth epithelial surface to regrow.) Keeping the epithelium intact speeds the healing process considerably. In addition, with LASIK there is less chance of post-procedure pain.

Preparing for LASIK

If you read this chapter immediately after reading Chapter 6, you will see that preparing for LASIK and preparing for PRK are almost identical. The important differences between the experience of LASIK and the experience of PRK happen during the procedure itself and in the recovery period.

As with PRK, you must refrain from contact lens wear prior to LASIK. In general, this means no soft lens wear for 2–3 days, and no rigid lens wear for 2–3 weeks before your LASIK.

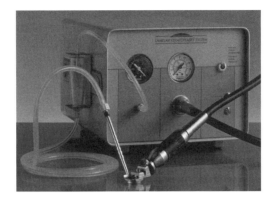

Figure 1 *The microkeratome is a device used to create a flap that, when turned back, exposes the stroma on which the laser works. (Photo of Moria microkeratome, courtesy of i-med pharma, Inc.)*

As with PRK, there are almost no restrictions on what you can eat or drink on the day of your LASIK, but do not consume alcohol or anything else that will make you drowsy for the procedure. Women should avoid makeup for the day. Take the medications that you normally take, but make sure that your ophthalmologist knows what you are taking before the surgery.

It is perfectly appropriate—in fact, it's a good idea—to bring a companion with you to the center. If you have to drive home, be sure you have someone who can do it for you. You will want to dress comfortably and casually, as you will remain in your street clothes for your LASIK.

At the Center

Except for the few minutes in which the procedure is taking place, coming in for a LASIK is much like coming in for a PRK. The whole process can take as little as an hour or hour and a half, but leave yourself some extra time. Most of the time you will spend at the center is preparation for the procedure (and a little bit of waiting). The actual LASIK procedure, like a PRK, goes very quickly. As with PRK, be sure to schedule yourself so that you have nothing else to do that day after you leave the center.

A routine much like the routine with PRK is followed for LASIK. Let us walk through a LASIK the way you would experience it at the Bochner Eye Institute.

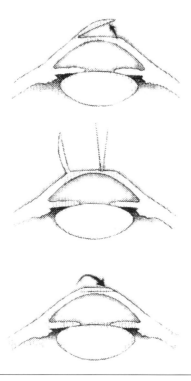

Figure 2 *The flap is created and lifted back, after which the laser ablates the exposed stroma. When the ablation is done (often in about a minute), the flap is replaced. (From Stein HA, Cheskes, AT, Stein RM:* The Excimer: Fundamentals and Clinical Use. *Thorofare, NJ, Slack, Incorporated, 1997. Reprinted with permission.)*

When you arrive at the center you will be greeted, checked in, and shown the facility (if you haven't seen it before). You will be encouraged to ask questions about anything that interests or concerns you.

Any final testing that needs to be done will be taken care of at this time. You'll also have a chance to meet with your ophthalmologist. He will give you an overview of the procedure and ask if there is anything else you wish to know about it. (Later, when you are in the laser suite, he will talk to you during the procedure to explain what is happening and guide you through each step.)

Preparing for LASIK

A half hour before your LASIK, you will be given pre-procedure medications. This will be a series of eye drops consisting of: an *antibiotic* to prevent infection; an *anti-inflammatory* to limit swelling and promote healing; and an *anesthetic* to numb your eye completely for the procedure (which will be entirely painless).

Shortly afterwards you will be taken into the laser room. A technician will see that you are positioned comfortably in the chair by the laser. The eye that is not being treated (or the eye that will be treated second) will be covered. At this point, the surgeon will usually enter the room. He will greet you again and explain to you step-by-step what is happening as the procedure begins.

LASIK

Since LASIK does not require the removal of epithelium, the first step is the creation of the flap. At the start, your ophthalmologist will put in an eyelid holder to prevent blinking during the procedure. Then he will make a few very light markings on the eye with a dye pencil or marker. These help him and make it easier to get the flap repositioned perfectly at the end of the procedure.

Then he will place the microkeratome on your eye. The microkeratome is held to the white of your eye by suction, so the first thing your ophthalmologist will do is position the base of the instrument, a suction ring, on the eye. When he is ready, suction will be turned on. Suddenly, your vision will go black. This is a good sign—it means the suction is working properly. Your ophthalmologist will then attach the microkeratome head to the ring. The microkeratome will automatically make a flap (a process that takes approximately 3 seconds).

Your ophthalmologist will now remove the microkeratome and proceed to the laser ablation. The ablation is almost precisely the same as it would be in PRK. (The ablation follows the refractive principles outlined in Chapter 5.) As in PRK, you will hear the laser make a clicking sound (sometimes a loud clicking sound). You will also probably notice the characteristic odor produced when the laser vaporizes tiny amounts of tissue.

In most cases, the laser portion of the procedure lasts just a few minutes (and often less than a minute). How long the laser procedure lasts depends on the correction needed. The more correction needed, the longer the procedure will take.

As in PRK, you will be asked to keep your gaze fixed on the blinking light. This can be more challenging in LASIK than in PRK, but you can do it. There is nothing to worry about here. A little bit of eye movement isn't a problem; and if there is too much movement, the surgeon can stop the laser and give you a moment to get readjusted.

"I felt blind without glasses or contacts."

NAME:	Shari Paulson
AGE:	38
OCCUPATION:	Salesperson in Florida
PROCEDURE:	Bilateral LASIK for myopia
OPHTHALMOLOGIST:	Performed at the Bochner Eye Institute
BEFORE LASER VISION CORRECTION:	Right eye: Unable to count fingers more than 5 feet distant Left eye: 20/400
AFTER LASER VISION CORRECTION:	Right eye: 20/25 Left eye: 20/15 (2 weeks after LASIK)

I flew all the way from Florida to Toronto to have laser vision correction because of the reputation of the Bochner Eye Institute. I went with five friends, and they all watched the procedure. Two of them had already been successful patients at the Bochner Eye Institute. After the procedure we went on a mini vacation in Toronto.

I think the most uncomfortable part is when they open your eye extremely wide with the lid holder. But then during the actual procedure, you don't feel anything. It's odd, thinking about what's happening to your eye and not feeling anything. It's over very quickly.

I haven't seen any halos. I haven't had any problems with night vision yet, though my vision is not perfectly clear. It's only been two weeks since I had the procedure. I went back to work that Monday, five days after. I don't need glasses or contacts anymore. I keep thinking I have contacts in. My optometrist says the results are good. The flap looks really good.

I was basically blind without glasses or contacts. It was a

drag to search for my glasses every morning. It was a hassle to be dependent on contacts or glasses to see at all. It has been nice to be able to wake up and see the alarm clock, to be able to just get up. Sometimes I forget, I think I have my contacts in. That's been really nice, that freedom.

Stopping to rest for a second to get one's gaze re-fixed is normal and no cause for concern.

Once the laser ablation is over (usually in a minute or so), all that remains is for the ophthalmologist to reposition the flap, make sure the repositioned flap is smooth, and satisfy himself that all is well with your eye. At this point, with the procedure just finished, in some centers patients will be asked if they want to read the eye chart. While their vision 2 minutes after LASIK isn't anywhere near as good as it will be a few days or a month later, many patients who have never before been able to read the eye chart without glasses are delighted by their new-found ability to see without correction.

Before you leave, you will be given a clear plastic eye shield. This is for you to wear to bed during the five nights following the procedure, so your eye(s) will be protected while you sleep. You can secure the shield to your eye(s) with regular (Scotch) tape. The entire LASIK procedure usually takes 10–15 minutes per eye. Most people (but not all) have both eyes done at the same time, one right after the other.

The LASIK Recovery Period

After LASIK, the corneal flap is held tightly to the eye by natural suction. Epithelium, which had been cut at the edges of the flap, regrows in about 24 hours. (Epithelial healing is faster than in PRK because much less is done to the epithelium during LASIK.) After LASIK, you should not rub your eyes, as this might disturb the flap. Blinking normally, however, will have no effect on the flap.

During the immediate post-LASIK period, it's a good idea to simply rest and take it easy. Sleep promotes healing, and you would be well advised to sleep as much as possible in the day or two after LASIK. The activity restrictions following LASIK are much the same as those after PRK:

- Don't swim or use whirlpools or hot tubs for the first week.
- For the first few days, close your eyes in the shower to keep soap and water out.
- For the first week, refrain from using eye makeup and avoid dusty environments or activities (like gardening) where you might get dirt or grit in your eyes.
- Smoking won't injure your eyes, but you may find it irritating for a day or two after LASIK.
- Don't drive until you are certain that your vision is good enough to allow you to do so safely.

LASIK patients often find their vision returns very quickly. Although it is not optimal, many LASIK patients return to work within a day or two.

LASIK Follow-up

After LASIK, it's very important to keep the follow-up appointments with your eye doctor. A typical follow-up schedule after LASIK will begin one day after the procedure, with additional visits at one week, one month, and later dates as recommended by your managing physician.

If the LASIK procedure doesn't deliver precisely the desired visual correction, it's a simple matter for the ophthalmologist to lift the flap and do a small laser enhancement. "Touching-up" is easy with LASIK. In fact, at the Bochner Eye Institute, we offer free enhancements for both LASIK and PRK patients. Other quality laser centers do this as well.

Comparing LASIK to PRK

LASIK and PRK are both excellent procedures. LASIK is a bit more challenging for the ophthalmologist, and scientific studies so far show that it carries a slightly greater chance of complications (because the flap adds a little bit of complexity to the procedure). However, LASIK is newer than PRK, and as the number of cases grows, the small difference in results should disappear.

In general, LASIK tends to be the preferred procedure for high degrees of myopia, and PRK is preferred for very low myopes. From the patient's perspective, LASIK tends to cause less pain and to have a shorter recovery period. There are, however, sometimes reasons related to your refractive error or to your ocular health that makes either PRK or LASIK the only good alternative for you. Your eye doctor can provide invaluable help in the decision process.

CHAPTER 8

Alternatives to Laser Vision Correction

Introduction

In the medical world, laser vision correction is considered an *elective* procedure. That means that people have laser vision correction because they want it rather than because they need it. People choose it because they perceive laser vision correction to be better than the alternatives.

Some of the alternatives, like glasses and contact lenses, are already familiar to you, perhaps too familiar. Virtually everyone who is considering laser vision correction has worn glasses, and most have tried contact lenses as well. Reviewing these familiar vision correction devices, along with some other alternatives, will help put laser vision correction into a useful perspective.

Glasses

Eyeglasses date from the middle ages, when they were used by monks to help them read and write. Today, a pair of glasses is an easily obtained, relatively low-maintenance vision correction device. Glasses can be inexpensive (although it's easy to spend quite a bit of money for a good-looking pair of fashion-conscious glasses).

From a medical standpoint, glasses are the safest means of vision correction. Glasses are a completely *non-invasive* technology, which means that they do not touch or change the eye in any way.

Disadvantages of glasses include:

- Many people are unhappy with how they look in glasses.
- Glasses can get in the way of sports and other recreational activities.
- Glasses are cumbersome for some otherwise simple activities, like using a camera or taking a walk in the rain.
- Some people are bothered by their dependence on glasses. For ex-

ample, people with strong prescriptions often worry about what they would do if there were an emergency and they couldn't find their glasses.

- Glasses are easily broken.
- Peripheral vision is often limited with glasses.

Contact Lenses

Contact lenses solve some of the problems that come with glasses. For example, contact lenses eliminate the cosmetic problems of glasses. Contacts also allow good peripheral vision and are preferred for sports and most recreational activities.

Because contact lenses rest directly on the eye, we cannot say that they are a truly non-invasive technology. However, contact lenses are *reversible*. In medical terms, a reversible procedure is one where it's possible to go back to the prior condition. Thus, when you take contact lenses off, the eye returns quickly to its normal, uncorrected state. For the most part, the eye is unchanged by contact lens wear. Contact lens wear is, therefore, like glasses, a reversible mode of correction.

Contact lenses also have some drawbacks:

- Most contact lenses require daily cleaning and disinfection.
- Contact lenses can be uncomfortable for people with dry eyes (and eyes inevitably get drier as we get older).
- Presbyopia and high degrees of astigmatism can be difficult to correct with contact lenses.
- Even after years of successful wear, an allergic or a toxic reaction to a contact lens (or lens care solution) can set in and make lens wear difficult or impossible.
- Contact lenses increase the wearer's risk of eye infection. In fact, the risk of ocular infection is greater with contact lens wear than with laser vision correction! Some contact lens-related infections can be very serious—they can even result in blindness or the loss of the eye.

Orthokeratology

A procedure that involves wearing a graded series of rigid contact lenses to gradually "reshape" the cornea, orthokeratology is useful only to treat low degrees of myopia. Most of the risks and drawbacks of contact lenses apply to orthokeratology.

In addition, to get a lasting effect from orthokeratology, one has to wear so-called "retainer" lenses on an ongoing basis. Continued follow-up visits to your eye doctor are also required. If you stop wearing

"I could read things for the first time in my life."

NAME:	Ross Skene
AGE:	46
OCCUPATION:	Music teacher, actor, musician
PROCEDURE:	LASIK for hyperopia and astigmatism
OPHTHALMOLOGIST:	Performed at the Bochner Eye Institute
BEFORE LASER VISION CORRECTION:	20/400
AFTER LASER VISION CORRECTION:	20/20

I first had to wear glasses when I was about 10 years old. I was one of the kids with Coke-bottle glasses.

I started wearing contact lenses when I was 19 and working as an apprentice actor. When soft contacts first came out I couldn't wear them because of my prescription. Most people with astigmatism have a problem getting whatever the latest eye thing is—it doesn't apply to them.

If you get a piece of dirt behind a hard contact lens, it's agony. I'm one of those people who could wear them 16 hours or more every day. I'm in my mid-forties now and they were tiring my eyes out.

The thing that really motivated me to try the laser procedure was that a company came out with a new soft contact lens, which was supposedly for people with astigmatism, and once again, because of my prescription, I couldn't wear that lens.

It was getting close to the point where I wouldn't be able to drive. Then I thought, well what are my options, and is it worth the risk? When I went to the Bochner Eye Institute at the recommendation of my optometrist, they explained all the risks to me. I had moments of apprehension, but they answered all my questions and concerns. They made me feel comfortable.

My wife came down with me and watched the whole operation. The assistant was wonderful. She talked me through the whole procedure. That helped a great deal.

I came home and I had quite a bit of burning in my eyes, the kind of burning sensation you get if you fall asleep with contact lenses in or if you get something behind one of them. We phoned the Institute, and they said to take the Tylenol III they had given me. I needed something just to get me over that little bit of pain. I finally took [the analgesic] and I fell asleep for 4 hours. I woke up, I looked out the window and I saw perfectly. I could read things for the first time in my life.

the "retainer" lenses, the cornea will slowly go back to its normal state, and the effect will be lost. Orthokeratology is a moderately invasive, reversible procedure.

Radial Keratotomy

Radial keratotomy (RK) involves using a diamond-bladed knife to make 4 or 8 incisions in a spoke-like (radial) pattern on the cornea (Figure 1). These incisions go to 90% of the corneal thickness, much deeper than either a PRK or LASIK ablation. RK incisions do not extend into the visual axis, where they would interfere with vision. (The "visual axis" is the central portion of the cornea through which we see.)

RK is an invasive, non-reversible procedure. Although RK can give good results, it is far less precise than laser vision correction. While some RK is still being performed, it is now being replaced by laser PRK and LASIK.

"ALK"

Automated lamellar keratoplasty (ALK) is a procedure that uses a

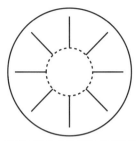

Figure 1 *Radial keratotomy incisions are made on the cornea around a central "clear zone."*

microkeratome (see Chapter 7) to both create a corneal flap and then to shape the stromal tissue below. Afterwards, the flap is closed and the eye heals quickly.

A non-reversible, highly invasive procedure, ALK was used largely to treat high degrees of myopia and hyperopia. Now that laser vision correction is available for this, ALK is rapidly becoming a thing of the past. Laser vision correction is far more precise than ALK.

KeraVision Ring

In this technique, two tiny arcs of plastic are implanted in the cornea, outside the visual axis. Because the ring segments are implanted in the cornea, the procedure is considered invasive. However, the segments can be removed; and evidence indicates that, when they are removed, the cornea returns to a condition very much like its original state. As a result, the technique is considered reversible.

At this point, this technique is useful only for correcting low to moderate degrees of myopia. However, studies on using similar techniques to correct hyperopia and astigmatism show promise. It remains to be seen whether the procedure is as precise as laser vision correction. KeraVision Ring implantation is performed in Europe and Canada; the U.S. Food and Drug Administration is still studying the technique for use in the U.S.

Intraocular Techniques

All of the surgical vision correction techniques we have discussed so far (including LASIK and PRK) are done at the surface of the eye. Intraocular techniques, as the name implies, are done within the eye. Two intraocular techniques hold promise: *phakic intraocular lenses* and *clear lens extraction.*

Intraocular techniques are derived from cataract surgery. (Cataracts are opacities in the crystalline lens that usually occur with age.) In modern cataract surgery, the crystalline lens is removed and replaced with a clear artificial lens called an *intraocular lens* (IOL). Many millions of cataract procedures are done every year around the world, so the technique has been greatly refined. Most ophthalmologists are skilled in cataract removal and IOL implantation.

Until recently, the crystalline lens was removed only when cataracts were present. Then some surgeons realized that the crystalline lens could be removed and replaced with an IOL as a way to correct refractive errors in eyes without cataracts. This technique is called *clear lens extraction* (CLE). The term "clear lens" applies because the crystalline lens that is removed has no opaque cataracts in it.

CLE is being studied in cases of very high degrees of myopia, where LASIK and PRK are less effective. (PRK is effective with low and moderate myopia. LASIK is effective with low, moderate, and high myopia. But neither LASIK nor PRK is optimum for extreme myopia.)

The phakic IOL technique is similar to clear lens extraction in that an aritificial lens is implanted in the eye. However, with a phakic IOL, the patient's crystalline lens is not removed. (The Greek word *phakos* means "lens"; and a person who has a crystalline lens is said to be "phakic"; a person whose crystalline lens has been removed, usually due to cataracts, is said to be "aphakic.") In the phakic IOL procedure, an IOL is implanted just in front of the crystalline lens. (One company refers to its phakic IOL as an "implantable contact lens.")

The advantage of the phakic IOL is that, in younger patients, the crystalline lens remains, and the patient doesn't lose the ability to accommodate (see Chapters 3 and 4). Because the crystalline lens is required for accommodation, CLE, which removes the lens, will end the patient's ability to accommodate.

Both CLE and phakic IOLs hold promise for patients with extreme refractive errors. LASIK and PRK, the standard treatments for the vast majority of refractive errors, are less effective for extreme refractive errors. For the great bulk of refractive errors, however, laser vision correction is more precise than CLE or phakic IOL implantation. Laser vision correction is also safer, easier, and far less invasive. To some degree, phakic IOL implantation is a reversible technique. CLE, however, definitely isn't. Once the crystalline lens is removed, nothing can replace it.

As good as phakic IOLs and CLE promise to be, their usefulness is likely to be limited to treating extreme refractive errors.

Laser Thermokeratoplasty

Laser thermokeratoplasty (LTK) uses a holmium:YAG laser (a different kind of laser from an excimer laser) to treat hyperopia. In LTK, the laser energy interacts with the corneal collagen (outside the visual axis), creating heat and causing the collagen fibers to contract. This has the effect of steepening the cornea and correcting the hyperopia.

LTK is a new technique that shows some promise but isn't yet proven. An invasive, nonreversible technique, caution is warranted. So far, LTK has been shown most effective with low degrees of hyperopia, where LASIK and PRK are also quite effective.

Putting Refractive Techniques in Perspective

Laser vision correction is obviously more invasive than either glasses or contact lenses; but compared to other surgical vision correction techniques, laser vision correction is relatively noninvasive. Laser vision correction is also substantially more precise than any other surgical vision correction technique currently available. This is the case because no other technique has a tool as precise as the excimer laser.

Laser vision correction is also very quick. PRK is done in 5–10 minutes. LASIK takes only a few minutes more. Most important, laser vision correction is a "mainstream" technique. Millions of laser vision correction procedures have already been done. It is now clear that, in the years to come, tens of millions more will be done.

Compare this to the other techniques. RK was useful in its day and is still effective in limited situations. However, there is nothing that RK can do that laser vision correction techniques can't do at least as well. RK is now disappearing. Similarly, ALK has been just about completely replaced by more precise laser techniques.

The KeraVision Ring, LTK, and intraocular techniques are all new technologies that are still under study. At most, a few hundred to a few thousand cases have been done with these new techniques, whereas several million laser ablation procedures (LASIK and PRK) have been done. Intracorneal rings, LTK, and intraocular techniques promise to be useful for treating a limited range of refractive errors in the future. In contrast, laser vision correction is capable of treating a broad range of refractive errors and is fully established today.

CHAPTER 9

The Decision Process

Many people first hear about laser vision correction from stories on radio and television. What prompts them to investigate further, however, is hearing about it again from a friend or acquaintance. More than anything else, the growth of laser vision correction is due to word-of-mouth from people who have experienced laser vision correction for themselves.

Word-of-mouth is a very powerful engine of growth. As we write this, in some parts of the United States the number of laser vision correction procedures has started to grow at almost 10% per *month*. At that rate, the number of laser vision correction procedures performed will more than double every year. At some point, of course, the excitement will subside, and laser vision correction will join glasses and contact lenses as one more accepted way of correcting vision.

But that time hasn't yet come. We are now in a transition period in which laser vision correction is generating excitement and enjoying rapid growth. The timing makes sense. Laser vision correction has turned an important corner and has gone from an experimental to a "mainstream" technique. There is no longer any question that laser vision correction works and works beautifully. People are overcoming their worries and starting to say "Yes" to laser vision correction.

The Key Is Understanding

What does it take for people to say "Yes" to laser vision correction? That question can be answered with a single word: "understanding." When people understand that laser vision correction can give them good natural vision and that the procedure is safe and effective, they opt for it readily. The hurdle is building that understanding.

Now that the researchers and scientists have created laser vision correction and demonstrated that it is safe and effective, it is up to practitioners like ourselves to educate the public. That's an important responsibility, and it is one of the reasons we wrote this book. We are confident that when people know the facts about laser vision correction, many will want it. Laser vision correction isn't for everybody; but for people who want to lessen their dependence on glasses and contact lenses, laser vision correction is a boon that brings freedom and happiness to their lives.

Since understanding is the key to reducing the fear that holds people back from laser vision correction, the Bochner Eye Institute, like many other laser centers, has created a process to help people learn about this new technology. Imagine for a moment that you are someone who is interested in laser vision correction and have come to us for information. In the remainder of this chapter, we'll walk you through the process of information gathering and decision making as it takes place at the Bochner Eye Institute.

When You Call

When you call the Bochner Eye Institute's special laser vision correction phone number (416-960-2020 or toll free 800-665-1987), your call will be picked up by a trained laser vision coordinator. This is a person whose primary job function is to teach people about laser vision correction. When you call, the laser vision coordinator will respond to your questions and invite you to come in for a personal consultation or a seminar on laser vision correction.

The Bochner Eye Institute's free seminars and one-on-one consultations offer a perfect learning opportunity. In addition to the laser vision coordinator, an ophthalmologist who does laser vision correction is present.

You will have plenty of opportunity to ask questions of our laser vision coordinator, the ophthalmologist, and perhaps a person who has recently experienced laser vision correction. You will have a chance to see what a laser facility is like. At the end of the seminar or consultation, you will be given additional information to take home and consider.

We always invite you to bring a friend. Since choosing laser vision correction is an important decision, many people want to talk it over carefully with a close friend or loved one. We encourage this, and we go one step further. We realize that, if the person with whom you discuss laser vision correction is to help you reach a major decision, he or she must know as much about laser vision correction as you do! So we invite your spouse or other support person to come not just to the seminar or consultation, but to accompany you every step of the way.

"They managed to give me confidence."

NAME: Angela Cameron
AGE: 38
OCCUPATION: Owns a funeral home
PROCEDURE: PRK for myopia and astigmatism
OPHTHALMOLOGIST: Dr. Harold Stein
BEFORE LASER VISION CORRECTION: 20/400
AFTER LASER VISION CORRECTION: Right eye: 20/20
Left eye: 20/15

My work as a funeral director puts me out in public. Even little things, like going from outside into a mausoleum, cause glasses to fog up, and at a funeral it's embarrassing to have to take your glasses off and wipe them. The surgery has given me a tremendous amount of freedom. I get many fewer headaches. I have sinus problems, and the bridge of my nose is very small. There was nothing worse than having a migraine and having to wear glasses. I just felt like taking them off to relieve the pressure a little. I've worn glasses all my life, and I was never happy, even with the vision that I got with them.

I wanted to get away from contact lenses and glasses. I wanted the visual comfort of being able to see peripherally and the freedom of not having glasses fog up. When you're giving your kids a kiss they're always falling off. I couldn't participate in sports.

For years I wore contacts comfortably, and then I just changed. My eyes started to get really dry, and they just didn't seem to tolerate the lenses anymore. I'd leave them out for six months and try again, and they just weren't comfortable. I've had every imaginable problem with contact lenses.

I went for a consultation with Dr. Harold Stein on a

Wednesday afternoon. And then I had laser vision correction done Thursday morning. I'm thrilled I had it done. They did a wonderful job, and I can't say enough about the staff. I was very nervous going into it, and they were just fabulous. I'm an exceptionally nervous person, and they managed to give me, of all people, the confidence to do it.

I find that people always say what's holding them back is the money, but I don't think it is. I think it's the fear of doing it. But from my perspective, it's quite reasonable. It's your eyesight. No vacation you could ever go on or anything you could buy could compare to having clear vision, forever.

It really feels like a miracle. We went on a vacation a few weeks ago, and I went in the ocean and I body surfed. And there are no more dents in my nose and no more foggy glasses. I'm thrilled with the outcome. The better-than-normal vision was a real bonus—I wasn't expecting to be corrected that well. I would definitely do it again, and I've encouraged a lot of my friends and people that I know to do it.

Going The Next Step

If you like what you hear and think that laser vision correction is possibly for you, you can make an appointment for a screening with a doctor. We'll test your vision and examine your eyes to make sure that you are a candidate for laser vision correction. If we discover any reason why you may not be a candidate, that will be explained to you.

If you are a candidate, you will have a chance to meet again with a laser vision coordinator, who will explain the laser vision correction process to you in detail. Of course, we encourage your companion to accompany you. The two of you will be able to ask any questions that you wish.

Often at this point it is possible to meet and talk with an ophthalmologist who does laser vision correction. After gathering all this information, reading our brochures, and meeting the ophthalmologist, many people make the decision that laser vision correction is right for them. This is the moment at which they make the appointment for their procedure.

Other Ways to Learn

While many of our patients come to us through the process we've just described, many more come to us through a referral process called *comanagement*. Comanagement is an arrangement whereby ophthalmologists like ourselves who perform laser vision correction share the pre-procedure examination and post-procedure follow-up with another eye doctor, often an optometrist.

This process works extremely well. All of the people with whom we comanage are specially trained as laser vision correction comanagers. In most cases, the comanager is the patient's regular eye doctor. Therefore, the patient and doctor know each other, and a bond of trust exists. Comanagement works well for teaching about laser vision correction because, when a trusted figure like their eye doctor explains laser vision correction and recommends it, people listen.

Comanagement is also a great convenience for patients. Patients frequently travel a long distance to get to the laser center. (For example, patients come to the Bochner Eye Institute in Toronto from all parts of the United States and Canada, as well as from around the world.) In contrast to the laser center, which may be quite distant, their regular eye doctor is usually located near where patients live or work.

Comanagement allows you to see your regular doctor for the preliminary work-up and counseling. You would then come to the laser center only on the day of your procedure and, perhaps, the day after. All the rest of your follow-up visits would take place at your regular eye doctor's office.

As Common as Braces

Although laser vision is growing, it has not yet gotten close to the level of acceptance that glasses and contact lenses enjoy. But those of us who perform laser vision correction are confident it will get there!

Let us offer an analogy. Everyone understands that dental braces can straighten crooked teeth. In North America, braces are a normal part of growing up for many children. People know in advance that dental braces will work, and they don't worry that their children will be harmed by them. The use of braces is widespread. If you didn't wear braces yourself, surely you know several people who did. Everyone accepts braces as safe and effective. Braces have earned this status by having been around long enough for people to get used to them.

Laser vision correction is also safe and effective. Years of scientific research (and 2 million treated eyes) have proven it to be. Not only is it safe and effective, laser vision correction is also an infinitely faster and gentler process than wearing braces. Compare the technologies for a moment. Laser vision correction ablates a tenth or a twentieth of a millimeter of soft tissue in a matter of minutes or seconds. There is little or no pain, and after a brief recovery period, the laser vision correction process is finished. All that remains is a handful of brief follow-up visits. (The only exception is the small fraction of patients who opt to have a second procedure to enhance their result.)

Where laser vision correction is over in minutes, dental braces move teeth with glacial slowness. Braces are painful, restrictive, and embarrassing; they require hours in the orthodontist's chair and years in your mouth. If braces can gain widespread acceptance, it is only a matter of time until laser vision correction does as well. The key is understanding.

CHAPTER 10

Choosing a Refractive Surgeon

Introduction

Once you have decided that laser vision correction is right for you, the next step is to choose an ophthalmologist to perform the procedure. You should look to a team that has been a part of the revolutions taking place in eye care and which has demonstrated a lasting commitment to permanently ameliorating the vision, and the lives, of their patients.

The following are some simple criteria that will enable you to choose the ophthalmologist who will provide you with the best possible treatment:

- The *education and training* of the ophthalmologist.
- His or her *experience.*
- His or her *affiliations.* Is the ophthalmologist affiliated with a university or a teaching hospital?
- His or her *reputation and track record.* Do patients recommend him or her strongly? Is he or she established and well regarded in the community?
- The *cost* of the procedure. Most treatments aren't covered by insurance.
- The *variety of treatments* offered by the doctor or center.
- A crucial factor is *personality and rapport.* How comfortable do you feel discussing your vision with the doctor and staff? Do you feel confident working with them?

Education and Training

Like all doctors, ophthalmologists go through many years of rigorous training before going into practice. This training usually includes four years of college pre-medical training, four years of medical school, one year as an intern, and three years of training as an ophthalmology resident. A total of 12 years may seem like a lot, but it's only the *minimum* required to practice ophthalmology—many ophthalmologists who perform laser vision correction have additional years of training. An ophthalmologist who performs laser vision correction should have training in corneal surgery.

Experience

Experience is an important factor. The more procedures an ophthalmologist performs, the better he or she becomes at laser vision correction. Experience leads to mastery.

You should feel free to ask your ophthalmologist how many laser vision correction procedures he or she has performed. Keep in mind that a good microsurgeon or corneal surgeon can learn to perform LASIK in a short time.

Affiliations

Affiliation with a well-known teaching hospital, medical school, or research center is a good sign that an ophthalmologist is dedicated to keeping up with new technology and new procedures.

Reputation and Track Record

Consider the general reputation of the practice in the community it serves. A practice or center that has operated for a number of years and which has a reputation for quality treatment is a safe bet. Ask around.

A good way to evaluate an ophthalmologist is to speak with his or her patients. A good clinic or practice will be happy to provide you with the names of people who have received a treatment similar to the one you are considering, and many will allow you to observe a procedure for yourself or to attend an informative seminar. Most offer a one-on-one consultation free of charge for individuals considering laser vision correction.

Cost

Because laser vision correction is an out-of-pocket expense for the majority of patients, cost is a consideration. Laser vision correction is no different from most other purchases: more often than not, you get what you pay for.

A good practice will offer a lifetime enhancement policy. In the unlikely event that you require an enhancement of your vision or another form of long-term follow-up care, a practice or center with a proven stability and reputation provides assurance that this care will be available.

"The outcome has proven to be all that you promised— and more."

Dear Dr. Stein,

Three weeks after surgery and I'm writing to thank you again for introducing me to "life after lenses"!

The outcome has proven to be all that you promised—and more.

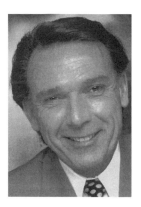

Not only was I able to return to the studio to write and present "First National" just a few hours after the operation, but there has also been noticeable improvement almost every day since. In fact, I've become so accustomed to my new sharpened vision, I've had to work hard to remember the "drops" schedule.

Please pass on my warmest regards—and thanks—to all the Bochner Eye Institute staff who made the experience such a pleasant one.

Sincerely,

Peter Kent
Global News
Toronto

Variety of Procedures Offered

A practice or a center which offers only one type of procedure might be inclined to direct you toward this procedure as the one that is best for you. Because they see the positive results of their work all day long, they'll naturally be inclined to emphasize those specific positive results. Consider consulting with a practice that offers different kinds of procedures for all types of vision, where doctors can pinpoint what is best for your eyes. No two eyes are alike.

Personality and Rapport

Before *any* procedure, it is of fundamental importance to be able to speak with the surgeon and to ask questions. You should expect to get an opinion directly from the person who treats your eyes. Excellent communication skills and the ability to foster trust are very important. When you are with the right surgeon, you will feel as if you are on the same wavelength and that your vision is in good hands.

Ophthalmologists are individuals. Each one brings a unique combination of experience, skills, personality, and level of candor to his or her relationships with patients. A particular treatment by a particular ophthalmologist that is perfect for your neighbor or your spouse might not be right for you. Ultimately, the best way to choose an ophthalmologist is to speak directly with him or her and ask the questions that are most important to you. You must feel confident that if a procedure is not appropriate for your condition, you will be told so.

You should expect total honesty and total candor from a good ophthalmic surgeon. The right surgeon will not push you in the direction of a particular procedure, but will present you with an unbiased assessment of your vision and the prospects of treatment based on the outcomes of previous patients who have had similar treatment. If you wish, you should be put in touch with individuals who have undergone treatment at his or her practice.

The Making of a Refractive Surgeon

How does a refractive surgeon come to be? Here are brief summaries of the authors' lives and work.

Dr. Harold Stein graduated from medical school in 1953. After completing an internship at Mount Sinai Hospital in Toronto, he received a fellowship to study ophthalmology and ophthalmic surgery at the prestigious Mayo Clinic in Rochester, MN, which he completed in 1957. He received a Master of Science degree from the University of

Minnesota, and he later became qualified as a plastic surgeon after study with world-renowned plastic surgeon Dr. Pomfret Kilner in England. In 1958, he began practicing in Toronto with his father-in-law, Dr. Maxwell K. Bochner, the founder of the Bochner Eye Institute. Dr. Stein spent ten years working side by side with Dr. Bochner and was soon recognized by the medical community for his expertise in cataract surgery, corneal transplants, and contact lenses. Over the years, he has been invited to speak at medical meetings and conferences throughout the world.

Dr. Stein is the author or co-author of 14 ophthalmology textbooks, many of which have gone into multiple editions. He is on the editorial board of several international ophthalmic journals and he has received honor awards from many distinguished international ophthalmic organizations. He has written over 200 articles for peer-reviewed medical journals. A full clinical professor at the University of Toronto Medical School, Dr. Stein is a pioneer in laser vision correction. Along with Dr. Cheskes and Dr. Raymond Stein, he was one of the first eye doctors in North America to practice laser vision correction.

Dr. Stein's commitment to the Toronto community extends beyond ophthalmology. He is an avid tennis player and is the co-author of *Hitting Blind: The New Visual Approach to Winning Tennis*. An amateur magician, he worked to preserve the memory of Harry Houdini by creating the Houdini Museum in Niagara Falls.

Dr. Albert Cheskes was a patient of Dr. Maxwell Bochner while growing up in Toronto. He graduated from the medical school of the University of Toronto in 1961. From 1963 to 1966 he trained at the Mayo Clinic as a resident in ophthalmology. He also received a Master of Science degree from the University of Minnesota. He is a widely-respected expert in cataract implant surgery, general ophthalmology, and ophthalmic surgery. Dr. Cheskes began to practice ophthalmology with Dr. Harold Stein and Dr. Bochner in 1966.

Throughout his career, Dr. Cheskes has been a pioneer in the field of ophthalmic surgery. He witnessed the first experiments with keratomileusis (an early form of corneal refractive surgery) in the early 1960's, and along with Drs. Harold and Raymond Stein was one of the first surgeons in Canada to perform laser vision correction procedures.

Dr. Cheskes is an assistant professor of ophthalmology at the University of Toronto, the Chief of Ophthalmology at Centenary Health

Center, and an active staff member at the Wellesley Division of St. Michael's Hospital in Toronto. He is also on the ophthalmology staff at Sunnybrook Hospital and Scarborough General Hospital.

Dr. Cheskes' son, Jordan, is currently in the third year of a five-year residency program in ophthalmology at the Mayo Clinic.

Dr. Raymond Stein is the son of Dr. Harold Stein and the grandson of Dr. Maxwell Bochner. He was a Benjamin Franklin Scholar at the University of Pennsylvania and graduated with honors from the University of Toronto Medical School in 1982. He did his residency in ophthalmology at the Mayo Clinic, and he was chosen for a prestigious one-year fellowship in corneal surgery at the Wills Eye Hospital in Philadelphia, PA. Dr. Stein is the author or co-author of six textbooks, as well as numerous chapters and scientific articles. He is the editor-in-chief of the international publication *Clinical Signs in Ophthalmology* and of the *Canadian Ophthalmic Case Consultation Journal.* He is a board member of the Canadian Society of Cataract and Refractive Surgery, and has received honor awards from the American Academy of Ophthalmology and the Contact Lens Association of Ophthalmologists. He is the Chief of Ophthalmology at Scarborough General Hospital and a cornea consultant for Mount Sinai Hospital. He is an assistant professor of ophthalmology at the University of Toronto.

Dr. Stein has been a medical director of the Bochner Eye Institute since 1987. He has also served as the medical consultant to the Beacon Eye Institute. A pioneer in laser vision correction with the excimer laser, he has performed over 10,000 PRK and LASIK procedures. He is an acknowledged expert in refractive surgery, corneal transplant surgery, and cataract surgery.

Dr. Stein has been a nationally ranked tennis player and a professional tennis instructor. He is the father of two daughters and of a son who is named after Dr. Maxwell Bochner.

The Bochner Eye Institute

Since its inception in 1929, the Bochner Eye Institute has been in the forefront of ophthalmology. Its founder, Dr. Maxwell K. Bochner (1900–1967), was also a founding member of Mount Sinai Hospital in Toronto and was chief of staff at both Mount Sinai and Scarborough General Hospital. A specialist in cataracts and diseases of the eye, Dr. Bochner was known for his careful and thorough diagnostic technique and is remembered for saving the eyesight,

"You were all terrific."

It is wonderful to see without glasses! The surgery was a piece of cake and I've been singing your praises! Bicycling is no problem. You were all terrific. Many, many thanks.

Valerie Pringle
CTV's *Canada AM*

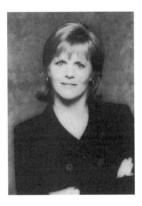

and the lives, of many people.

Today, Dr. Harold Stein, Dr. Albert Cheskes, and Dr. Raymond Stein are the medical directors of the Bochner Eye Institute. Together, they represent 85 years of experience as practicing ophthalmologists. The Bochner institute remains steadfast in its mission of providing the best possible eye care for its patients and the highest degree possible of communication between patient and care-provider. They strive to provide a level of caring and compassion for their patients modeled on Dr. Bochner's example. The directors and staff of the Bochner Clinic are proud to continue serving the Toronto area and beyond. Drs. Harold and Raymond Stein and Albert Cheskes regularly treat patients from all corners of the globe. Recognition of its leadership role in ophthalmic surgery and its commitment to excellence can be seen in the significant number of ophthalmologists who seek treatment there. The directors of the Bochner Eye Institute are regularly invited to speak and give seminars at meetings, clinics, and ophthalmic conferences around the world.

The commitment of Drs. Harold and Raymond Stein and Albert Cheskes to the future of the Bochner Eye Institute as well as the future of eye care is embodied in the recently opened Stein/Cheskes Laser Center of the Bochner Eye Institute. The laser center houses the latest technological advances in laser vision correction, including both a Nidek excimer laser and the VISX Star SmoothScan excimer laser, as well as viewing facilities for educational purposes, which also enable relatives and prospective patients to watch live procedures.

CHAPTER 11

Questions and Answers

Introduction

Our years of offering laser vision correction have brought us together with thousands of people looking for information about this exciting procedure. There are some questions that everyone wants answered; and there is some information that we, as ophthalmologists, would want every one of our patients to know in advance. We believe in having well-informed patients. The only surprise we want our laser vision correction patients to experience is the delight of good natural vision.

In this chapter we've collected the most frequently asked questions. Having them together in a group will save you from having to look each one up in its own chapter of the text.

How long does laser vision correction take?

The actual laser work itself usually takes less than a minute per eye. It can take a little longer or a little less, depending on the correction done. Including preparation time, you can expect that PRK will require 5–10 minutes per eye in the chair where the laser work is performed. LASIK will take just a bit longer, approximately 10–15 minutes per eye. Your office visit on the day of the procedure should take about an hour and a half. It's important to show up at the appointed time and leave the remainder of your day free. You won't be spending your whole day at the laser center, but it's very helpful to be able to simply rest and relax after the procedure. The time before the procedure will give you a chance to visit with your ophthalmologist and ask any last minute questions, as well as complete any testing that remains.

Does laser vision correction hurt?

There is no pain whatsoever during either the LASIK or PRK procedure. This is because analgesic (pain numbing) drops keep the eye from feeling anything at all while the operation is in progress. After the operation, LASIK patients may notice mild irritation. They may experience a little sensitivity to light and perhaps have some watering of the eyes for a day or two after the procedure. In terms of pain and recovery, LASIK is a mild procedure from which patients recover quickly.

PRK patients may experience mild discomfort for a few days following their procedure. Some PRK patients find there is no pain whatsoever, others find it minimal, and still others (about 10%) describe the post-operative pain as moderate. Patients who have pain usually describe it as feeling as if there were a lash or specks of dirt in their eye.

To reduce the chance of pain following PRK, a "bandage" contact lens is placed on the eye to protect it until the corneal epithelium can grow back over the cornea, beneath the contact lens. In addition, medication is used to prevent pain. If you experience pain after PRK, you can be given additional medication that should eliminate the problem. Once the surface of the cornea, the epithelium, has regrown—usually within 3 or 4 days—the pain, if there is any, should go away completely. Most PRK patients experience some sensitivity to light while the epithelium is growing back. They may also experience a burning sensation when putting in eye drops for the first 2 or 3 days after surgery.

Will I be awake during laser vision correction?

Yes, you will be awake and alert for PRK and LASIK. You may even be asked to assist in aligning the laser for the procedure by keeping your gaze fixed on a blinking red light.

I'm farsighted. Can laser vision correction help me?

Yes. Once limited to nearsighted people, laser vision correction can now help people who are nearsighted, farsighted, or have astigmatism. There are some limitations—for example, laser vision correction may not be the procedure of choice for eyes with extreme refractive errors. Today, however, laser vision correction is capable of correcting most people's refractive error.

Will I need glasses after laser vision correction?

The great majority of laser vision correction patients do not need glasses for normal distance vision tasks (like sports or driving). Some people *choose* to wear glasses after laser vision correction in order to

Race Driver Goes Faster

NAME:	Ludwig Heimrath
AGE:	63
OCCUPATION:	Professional Race Car Driver
PROCEDURE:	PRK for hyperopia and astigmatism
OPHTHALMOLOGIST:	Dr. Raymond Stein
BEFORE LASER VISION CORRECTION:	20/400
AFTER LASER VISION CORRECTION:	20/25

If you have glasses in a race car and the weather is bad, say fog or rain, the heat in the race car will make the glasses fog up, and there's not much you can do about it. That problem is eliminated now that I don't have to wear glasses. I'm quite happy with that. I go faster in the same car since I had the proce-
dure done. I wasn't expect-ing that to hap-pen. There's a definite change in my lap times since I had my vision cor-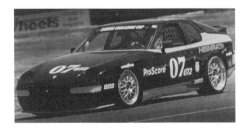rected. After my laser vision correction, I won the Cana-dian Racing Championship. I owe my recent driving suc-cess to my restored vision.

I never wore contact lenses. I tried them once and I hated them. They irritated my eyes. I wore glasses for about 25 years. I knew of three or four very famous drivers who had their vision corrected with lasers: Emerson Fitipaldi and Paul Tracy, for example. I talked with Emerson Fitipaldi, and he said it was great.

I had my left eye done first. If I could do it again, I would have both eyes done at the same time. My vision took a few weeks to become perfect, but I noticed the difference immediately after the procedure. In fact, they told me not to drive home, but I did. I drove home without glasses. I didn't need a chauffeur. And my eyes got better every day after that.

I didn't experience any pain. I didn't take any pain killers. My eyes didn't water. My eyes healed flawlessly. The Bochner Eye Institute gets a lot of customers out of me because people notice that I don't wear glasses anymore. I've recommended this procedure to many, many people. I think it's the best way to go.

One amazing thing is that my near vision got better, as well as my far vision. I can read things without glasses that I couldn't read before. That wasn't supposed to happen, but I'm glad it did.

get the sharpest possible vision or to help with demanding visual tasks, like driving at night.

People in their mid-40s and older who have good distance vision in both eyes will need correction for reading. This is an entirely normal condition called *presbyopia* and has nothing to do with laser vision correction. After a certain age, *everyone* who has excellent distance vision will need some kind of correction for reading. From about age 45 onward, the only people who can read without glasses are people who are slightly nearsighted, and they can't see clearly at distance!

If you are over 40 and, after discussion with your doctor, would like to have glasses-free vision at both distance and near, laser vision correction can correct one eye for distance vision and the other eye for near vision. This is a technique called *monovision.* Many people over 40 find monovision highly satisfactory, but it is very important to discuss it carefully in advance with your eye doctor. If you are interested in monovision, you can try it out first with contact lenses. Ask your eye doctor for a trial.

Can I go blind from the laser?

This is an easy question. The answer is "No." No one has ever been blinded by the laser, and no one is ever likely to be. The excimer laser beam works on the very top-most layer of eye tissue that it strikes. Each successive pulse of the laser removes just a tiny amount of tissue from this top-most layer. No energy from the laser penetrates below the surface of the eye. This is what makes the excimer laser so safe!

That doesn't mean that nothing can go wrong during laser vision correction. There are risks, and you should be aware of them. However, being blinded by the laser isn't one of the risks.

Are there medical reasons why I might not be able to have laser vision correction?

Yes. Even if your refractive error is one that can be corrected by a laser procedure, there are some eye conditions and medical problems that could take you out of the running for laser vision correction. The list of conditions includes diabetic retinopathy, cataracts that produce loss of vision, severe dry eye, autoimmune disease (such as lupus or rheumatoid arthritis), uncontrolled glaucoma, and very large pupils. If for physical or psychological reasons you are unable to lie still and focus during the procedure, you may not be a candidate.

Some conditions may require that you postpone laser vision correction until they resolve. These include: unstable refraction (your glasses prescription keeps changing every year), pregnancy, and herpes infection.

This is why it is important that you consult with an eye doctor and get a thorough eye exam with a careful medical history prior to giving laser vision correction serious consideration.

Are there attitudes or lifestyle issues that should make me think carefully before embarking on laser vision correction?

Yes. If you absolutely need 20/20 or better vision for your job, or if you can't tolerate anything less than perfect vision in both eyes, then laser vision correction may not be for you. Similarly, you may not wish to have laser vision correction if you require absolutely perfect night vision or if you are unwilling or unable to commit to taking follow-up medications and coming in for follow-up visits. If any of these apply to you, be sure to talk to your eye doctor about them before going forward with laser vision correction.

Will laser vision correction help me get rid of my reading glasses?

Almost everybody 45 or older needs some sort of vision correction for reading. If your distance vision is fine, and if all you need glasses for is reading, laser vision correction is probably not for you. If, however, you are near- or farsighted *and* need reading glasses, there are two laser vision correction options. The first is to have both eyes corrected for distance. If you choose this option, you will have good functional distance vision but will need glasses or a contact lens in order to be able to read comfortably.

The alternative is to correct one eye for distance and the other for near. This is called *monovision*, and it works well for many people. However, monovision isn't for everybody. The best way to tell if monovision will work for you is to try it with contact lenses. Speak to your eye doctor about this. Now that disposable lenses are readily available, it's a simple matter to try monovision for a few days or a week to see if it works for you.

What are the risks of laser vision correction?

The chance of having a serious, vision-threatening complication as a consequence of laser vision correction is very low—far less than 1%. But the risk isn't zero, so it is important that you know the risks and be able to put them into perspective.

Infection To prevent infection, you will be given antibiotic drops both before and after the procedure. Post-operative infections are rare in PRK and extremely rare in LASIK. When they do occur, they tend to be minor and clear up quickly with treatment. However, a small chance of serious infection exists, and it is therefore important to take the prescribed medication as directed and come in for follow-up visits. If there is a problem after the procedure, don't hesitate to call your eye doctor!

Pain Some patients experience discomfort, particularly following PRK. This is easily treated with medication. Mild irritation, sensitivity to light, and watering of the eyes can be expected in the first few days after a PRK or LASIK procedure.

Undercorrection or overcorrection Some laser vision correction patients wind up with either a little more or a little less correction than desired. A laser enhancement procedure at a later date is usually all that is needed to take care of the under- or overcorrection.

"My world is brighter and more colorful."

NAME:	Oskar Johansson
AGE:	21
OCCUPATION:	Olympic-level sailor, engineering student
PROCEDURE:	PRK for myopia
OPHTHALMOLOGIST:	Performed at the Bochner Eye Institute
BEFORE LASER VISION CORRECTION:	Right eye: 20/80 Left eye: 20/200
AFTER LASER VISION CORRECTION:	20/20

Vision is crucial in sailing. In the Laser, the class of boat I sail, you're only about a foot off the water. Glasses are a real problem, waves splash constantly and you have to maintain focus. I wore contacts. That was also a problem, since I would wear them for up to eight hours at a time. Messing with en- zyme cleaners and other solutions takes time and concentration away from a regatta. I travel to lots of different places to race, and at some it's dif- ficult to find a location for preparing and put- 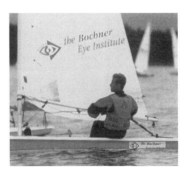 ting-in contacts. Sometimes there are only port-a-potties. With no place to take lenses out, my eyes could get very irritated.

I have a very tight schedule. I'm a full-time university stu- dent studying engineering, as well as training for the Olympics. In the autumn, especially, there's a limited amount of daylight. So the time spent hassling with contacts is a serious consideration.

I realized that in order to be competitive I would need to always have two good pairs of glasses, a pair of prescription sunglasses and two sets of contacts. It was going to be pretty expensive. My parents suggested laser vision correction.

I went for a free consultation with Dr. Harold Stein at the Bochner Eye Institute. I didn't have much time, since it was in May, and I was in between exams and a trip to Europe to race. I already felt very comfortable with the procedure after talking to one of my Canadian teammates, who has a sister who had the same procedure. Once the people at the Bochner Institute explained it to me, I asked if there were any cancellations. I had it done right away. I trusted Dr. Harold Stein.

Now I have basically perfect vision. I see halos at night sometimes, but that has gotten better with time. Having good vision is worth it. My world is brighter and more colorful. I hadn't realized it was a bit gray before. I didn't always keep my glasses clean. Now the colors are sharper. The procedure has made life much easier and my sailing has improved.

I would definitely recommend laser vision correction, and I highly recommend the Bochner Eye Institute. For me, especially, it's worth the money. I would have had to invest in a new pair of glasses and a new pair of contacts each year over the next 25 years, at least. Plus, I get all that time without the hassle of glasses and contacts. It's worth it for that alone—no glasses or contact lenses.

Loss of best corrected vision After laser vision correction, a few patients find they have lost a small amount of visual sharpness compared to their vision *with glasses* before their procedure. Usually this means a loss of the ability to read the bottom one to three lines on the eye chart. In some cases, patients regain this ability as the eye continues to return to normal during the year following their procedure.

Night vision problems In the weeks and months following laser vision correction, it is common to see halos or starbursts around bright objects at night. In most, but not all, cases this ceases to be a problem by 4 to 6 months after the procedure.

Haze Slight haze is a normal part of the healing reaction. Most patients are unaware of it, although sometimes, particularly after PRK, the haze is noticeable. Haze tends to resolve slowly over a period of several months. Medication can be used to speed the healing process.

Regression There is a small tendency for the laser-treated eye to return in the direction of its pretreatment state. Should this happen to you, you may need an enhancement (another laser procedure) to touch up the eye. Alternatively, you can wear a thin pair of glasses to sharpen your vision. For some patients, glasses for use in night driving are all that is needed to deal with a small amount of regression.

Unrealistic expectations One of the most serious risks of laser vision correction is disappointment based on unrealistic expectations. Nearly everyone who experiences laser vision correction greatly reduces his or her dependence on glasses or contact lenses; but no one can promise you in advance that laser vision correction will allow you to be free of glasses forever. Because the laser procedure primarily corrects distance vision, patients eventually need reading glasses (or monovision). Some laser vision correction patients will need a pair of glasses with thin lenses for critical tasks, like driving at night.

Is laser vision correction the same as RK?

No. RK (for "radial keratotomy") was an early (pre-laser) refractive surgery procedure. Developed by a Russian ophthalmologist, RK uses a knife to create 4 or more small incisions that reshape the corneal tissue. In contrast, laser vision correction uses a computer-controlled excimer laser to ablate corneal tissue either at the surface (for PRK) or just below the surface (for LASIK). A great advance in its time, RK taught ophthalmologists that, by changing the shape of the cornea, the quality of vision could be dramatically improved. Because it is far less precise than laser vision correction (and has other drawbacks), RK is rapidly being supplanted by laser techniques.

Should I have both eyes corrected at once?

Most people now decide to have both eyes corrected at the same "sitting." It was once thought that there was added risk, particularly of infection, if both eyes were done at once. But scientific research and the experience of tens of thousands of patients show that there is little additional risk when both eyes are corrected on the same day. It is also much more convenient to do both eyes at the same time.

Correcting your eyes at different times also means two trips to the laser center and two recovery periods. There would also be a period after the first procedure when one eye can see well, while the other eye still has its old refractive error. Many people find this imbalance in their eyes very unpleasant and decide to move up the date of their second procedure.

However, if you would be more comfortable doing the second eye after seeing the result with the first eye, the choice is entirely yours.

Glossary

Ablate To remove tissue by vaporizing it (as with a laser).

Accommodation The ability of the eye to change its focus from distant objects to near ones.

Astigmatism A refractive error in which the cornea (and/or the crystalline lens) has different curvatures in different meridians. The result is an inability to focus light on the retina.

Cornea The clear, dome-shaped central surface of the eye through which light enters. The cornea is not only the "window" that lets light into the eye, it is also part of the optical system that focuses light on the retina.

Crystalline lens The eye's natural lens. The crystalline lens is able to change shape and thereby change focus, allowing the eye to accommodate. (The ability to accommodate declines with advancing age.)

Bowmans layer The thin layer of cornea between the epithelium and the stroma.

Descemets membrane A thin layer of the cornea between the stroma and the endothelium.

Diopter A measure of the strength of a lens.

Endothelium (corneal endothelium) A single layer of cells on the inner surface of the cornea. The endothelium forms the border between the cornea and the inner eye.

Epithelium (corneal epithelium) The outermost corneal layer. The epithelium protects the cornea from the environment.

Hyperopia The condition of being farsighted. Hyperopic people ("hyperopes") have difficulty seeing close objects.

Intraocular lens (IOL) Small plastic lenses that are placed within the eye either following cataract surgery or in refractive surgery to improve vision in persons with extreme correction needs.

Iris The colored portion of the eye that controls the size of the pupil.

KeraVision Ring Tiny plastic arcs that can be implanted in the cornea to change its refractive power. Effective for nearsightedness, KeraVision Ring technology is being studied for hyperopia and astigmatism.

LASIK A laser vision correction procedure that uses a microkeratome to create a corneal flap. The laser then ablates tissue beneath the flap. At the end of the brief procedure, the flap is closed, and the eye heals quickly.

Microkeratome A device placed on the eye for producing a flap as part of the LASIK procedure.

Monovision A way of dealing with presbyopia in which one eye is corrected for distance and the other eye for near. This can be done with contact lenses or laser vision correction.

Myopia Nearsightedness. A condition in which the eye's optical system focuses light in front of the retina, causing distant images to appear blurred, while near objects may be clear.

Presbyopia A normal part of aging in which the eye loses the ability to accommodate.

PRK A laser vision correction technique in which the ocular surface is ablated directly.

Pupil The opening in the iris that allows light to enter the eye. The pupil responds to changes in the quantity of light, getting larger ("dilating") in low-light conditions.

Radial keratotomy A refractive surgery technique in which a diamond-bladed knife is used to make small radial cuts in the cornea. Effective only for correcting mild to moderate myopia, radial keratotomy is rapidly being supplanted by laser vision correction.

Refraction (1) the bending of light by a lens or optical system. (2) the process of measuring the eye's ability to focus.

Refractive error The inability to focus light properly on the retina. The common refractive errors are nearsightedness, farsightedness, and astigmatism.

Refractive surgery Ocular surgery that corrects refractive errors by reshaping the cornea or implanting a lens within the eye.

Retina The back portion of the eye on which light is focussed. The retina "translates" the image into nerve impulses that are sent to the brain for processing.

Stroma (corneal stroma) The "body" of the cornea, accounting for approximately 90% of corneal thickness.

Visual acuity Quality of vision, as measured by the ability to read a Snellen eye chart.

Index

20/20 vision 12, 25, 35
  Defined 23–24

Ablation
  Corneal 6
  Defined 38
Accommodation 21, 68
Alcohol 46, 56
"ALK" (automated lamellar
  keratoplasty) 66–67
Analgesic 50
Anesthetic 48,58
Antibiotic 48, 57
Anti-inflammatory 48,57
Aphakic 68
Astigmatism 2, 9, 10, 23, 27
  Correcting with laser surgery 41
  Defined 29–32
Autoimmune diseases 10, 11, 89

"Bandage" contact lens 50
Bifocal lens 3, 24
Bochner Eye Institute 12, 45, 46, 56,
81, 82–84
  Telephone number 72
Bochner, Maxwell K., MD 81, 82
Bowmans layer 20
Buzard, Kurt 2

Cataract surgery 1, 68
Cataracts 11, 68
Cheskes, Albert, MD 81
Clear lens extraction 68–69
Comanagement 75
Consultation 72
Contact lenses 3, 7, 12, 14, 23
  Before LASIK 55
  Before PRK 46
  Difficulties with 12, 14–15, 16
  For reading 21, 22, 32–35

Converging lens 18–19
  Defined 19
  To correct farsightedness 29, 30
Cornea 3, 18
  Diagram 20
  Refractive surgery and 21, 37–43
  Structure and function 19–21
Crystalline lens 18, 19, 27
  Surgery 21

Descemets membrane 20
Diopter 23, 25
Diverging lens 18, 22
  Defined 19
  To correct nearsightedness 27
Dry eye 11

Emmetropia 27
Endothelium, corneal 20
Enhancement (see "Touch-up"
  procedures)
Epithelium, corneal 20, 49
  LASIK and 42–43
  PRK and 41–42
Excimer laser 4, 6, 23, 38–40
Eye(s)
  Diagrams 17, 19
  Structure 17–19

Farsightedness 2, 3, 9, 10, 27
  Correction of 25, 32, 40
  Defined 28–29
  Diagram 29
  Extreme 6, 21
Fluctuating vision 52
Foyodorov, Svyatoslav 4
Franklin, Benjamin 3

Glasses (spectacles) 3, 7, 9, 10, 23,
63–64
  Difficulties with 12, 14–15, 16
  For reading 35

Glaucoma
　Uncontrolled 11, 89

Holmium:YAG laser 69
Hyperopia (see Farsightedness)

Infection 11
Intraocular lens (IOL) 6, 67–68
Intraocular techniques 67–68
Iris 21

KeraVision Ring 4, 67

Laser in situ keratomileusis (see LASIK)
Laser thermokeraoplasty (LTK) 69
LASIK 21, 55–62
　Defined 42–43
　Procedure duration 85
Lenses
　Measuring power of 22–23
Lupus 11, 89

Medications 46, 48, 57
Microkeratome 42, 55, 58
　Pictured 56
Micron
　Defined 41
"Miracle factor" 2
Monovision 12
　Defined 32–35
Myopia (see Nearsightedness)

Nearsightedness 2, 3, 4, 9, 10, 24
　Correction of 25, 29, 32
　Defined 27–28
　Diagram 28
　Extreme 6, 21
Night glare 52–53
"No line" lens (see Progressive lens)

Omnivision (see Monovision)
Optic nerve 18
Orthokeratology 64–66

Phakic intraocular lenses 67–68
Phakic clear lens extraction 68
Phoropter 32
Photorefractive keratectomy (see PRK)

Pregnancy 11
Presbyopia 12
　Defined 21–22
　Implications of 35
PRK 21, 45–54
　Defined 41–42
　Duration of 85
Progressive lens 32
Pupil 21
　Large pupil size 11, 89

Radial keratotomy (see RK)
Refraction
　Correcting with laser surgery 39–41
　Defined as corrective lens fitting
　　process 32
　Defined as optical term 19
Refractive error 27–35
　Defined 19
Retina 18, 22, 23
Rheumatoid arthritis 11, 89
RK (radial keratotomy) 4, 66

Seminars 72
Sensitivity to light 52
Smoking 54, 61
"Snellen acuity" 24
Snellen chart 24
Spectacles (see Glasses)
Stein, Harold, MD 80
Stein, Raymond, MD 82
Stroma 20
　During LASIK surgery 42–43
　During PRK surgery 41–42
Swimming 14, 53, 61

"Touch-up" procedures (enhancement)
54, 61
Trifocals 32

Visual acuity 24
　Measuring 25

Water sports 14